HEALTHY CHOICES
IN AN
UNHEALTHY WORLD

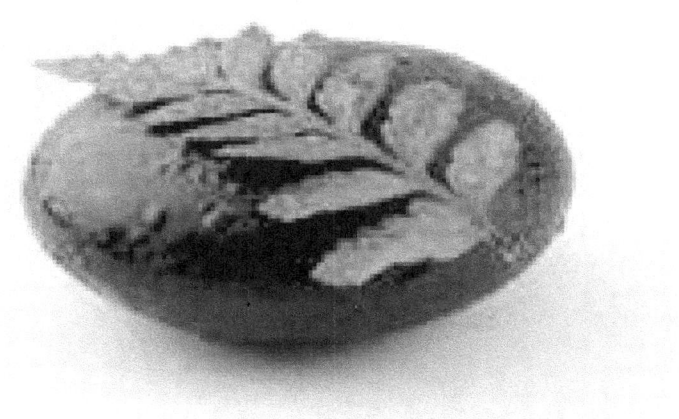

by
Sheila K. Miles
N.D., N.H.S.D.
edited by Justice Valentine

2011

DISCLAIMER

The health and nutrition information contained in this book is for educational purposes only. It is not meant to replace the advice of a medical professional.

Sheila K. Miles, N.D., N.H.S.D.
2011

To purchase this book,
go to
amazon.com
barnesandnoble.com
http://www.choosing-natural-health.com
or order through fine bookstores everywhere

Visit Dr. Miles' blog at
http://drsheilamiles.blogspot.com

Contact Dr. Miles at
drsheilamiles@hotmail.com

FORWARD

I began my natural health journey years ago. It really started when I was a child -- I was always the one who would "doctor" my dolls. Growing older, I decided to be a surgical nurse.

All my childhood, I watched my father suffer with rheumatoid arthritis in every joint. He would come home from work at night and fasten heating pads to his elbows and knees. The only options the doctors offered were steroids and pain medicine. At that time, gold shots were the treatment of choice, and his arthritis was so severe that he started on this dangerous course. Not long after that, he developed lung cancer. The doctors had no answer about the cause of arthritis or the cancer, or any treatment to make him better, and he passed away at the age of 50.

Mom suffered with horrible migraine headaches, sometimes for days at a time, with all the vomiting and everything that goes with them. These headaches seem to run in my family. My grandmother had them as well, and would temporarily go blind until the headache subsided. Once again, the doctors had no answer and no treatment.

Then I got married and "life" happened. My ambition to work in the medical field had to wait.

Eight years of marriage and one wonderful son later, I was facing a divorce and starting over. I still held onto my dream of the medical profession, but at this time it just wasn't possible to make a living, go to school, and have any time left for my son. So once again it was put on the back burner.

I re-married and had another son, along with a stepson. I had toxemia, as it was then called; now it is pre-eclampsia. Anyway, the result is the same. You usually deliver early, and it can be life-threatening. I'd had toxemia with my older son, too, but not as severely. I asked the doctor numerous times what caused it, and got the same reply: "We don't know -- some women just have it." I wasn't satisfied, but had to settle for it, at the time.

My new baby was born 10 weeks premature, and had some health problems, including asthma; as a matter of fact, both of my sons had asthma. I have always heard that people to learn from are sent to you, and I've had my share!

Time passed and the baby grew, then abruptly gave up his bottle. I was concerned about calcium, since I then thought milk was the only source. I asked his doctor if there was something else I could give him to supplement the calcium. She told me that they didn't really study nutrition in medical school, and didn't know what else I could do besides a multi-vitamin. She didn't say a word about green leafy vegetables, and at that time I didn't have a clue.

With two children who had asthma, our house became a "drug store." We had a good supply of inhalers and a nebulizer on standby, and when all else failed, we made a mad dash to the nearest hospital for even more drugs. Those drugs probably saved my children, but deep down inside I knew there had to be a better way.

My older son, who was about 12 at the time, took up Kung Fu, a form of Chinese martial arts. His teacher knew about Chinese medicine, so my son started using a few of their remedies. They worked! That was a time when natural remedies were virtually unheard of in this area, and I wasn't too sure about them, but I *was* interested.

I'd become very disillusioned with the medical profession, and was looking for something different. Here they were, with all their degrees but no answers for any of my family members. I didn't want my family tied to drugs for life. I just knew that, somewhere, there was something better.

One day, during my lunch break at work, I picked up a magazine and saw an article that piqued my interest. The author had just graduated college as a Naturopathic Physician. I had never heard of it, but she described exactly what *I* wanted to do. I made a few phone calls (no internet back then), and learned more about becoming a Naturopath. The more I found out, the more I wanted to do it.

I had geared my high school education toward nursing school, emphasizing chemistry and math. Then, after high school, I had enrolled in some classes at the local college. So, with my previous credits in hand, I went to work. It was an uphill battle, but I made it. My husband and my family were very supportive, and helped me so much along the way. In 2000, I graduated as a "Doctor of Naturopathy" and also a "Doctor of Natural Health Science." I started my new career!

Not surprisingly, arthritis, migraines, toxemia, cancer, and asthma became my pet peeves. I was bound and determined to find out the causes and anything that offered relief, and there are specific causes for all of these, and things that can help. I can't use the word "cure," because it offends the medical profession, but I can say that the remedies can make them 100% better.

Toxemia is one I think I've solved. I heard a theory that it can be caused by too much copper, which also causes numerous other health problems. So I did a hair analysis on myself, and my copper was through the roof. I tested other family members, and they had it, too.

I had to track down the source of this copper, since I had almost lost both of my babies. It took a while, but I found it. We had a well that we had used when I was growing up, and for the early part of my adult life. There was one copper fitting on one of the lines. The water from the well was soft water, which leaches out copper more quickly than hard water. This one copper fitting may have almost cost the lives of my two boys.

Arthritis, cancer, migraines, asthma and other major diseases are more difficult to solve, but they do have specific causes and can be treated to make your quality of life much better.

This book contains information about nutrition and other helpful things I've learned during my career, presented in what I hope is a way that almost anyone can understand without having to feel they're going back to school.

I hope you'll find something you've been looking for!

Sheila K. Miles, N.D., N.H.S.D.
http://drsheilamiles.blogspot.com
drsheilamiles@hotmail.com

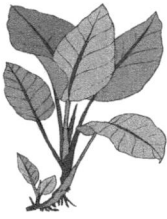

<u>HEALTHY</u> CHOICES
IN AN
UNHEALTHY WORLD

HEALTHY CHOICES in an UNHEALTHY WORLD

TABLE OF CONTENTS

HEALTHY CHOICES in an UNHEALTHY WORLD

TABLE OF CONTENTS, continued

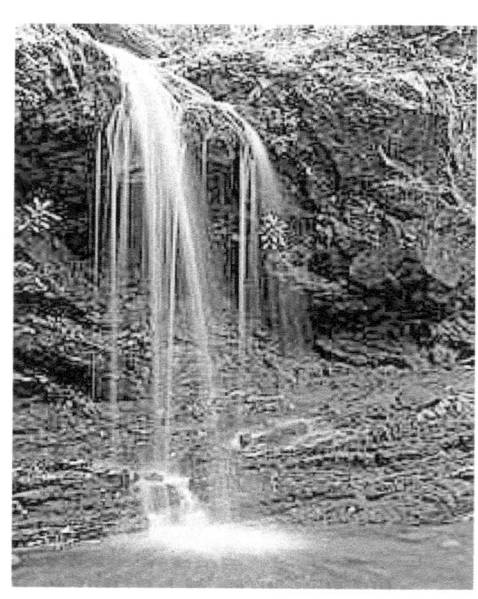

HEALTHY CHOICES
IN AN *UNHEALTHY* WORLD

CHAPTER 1
DIET

LOOKING FOR
HEALTH PROBLEMS
ON THE END
OF YOUR FORK!!

DIET

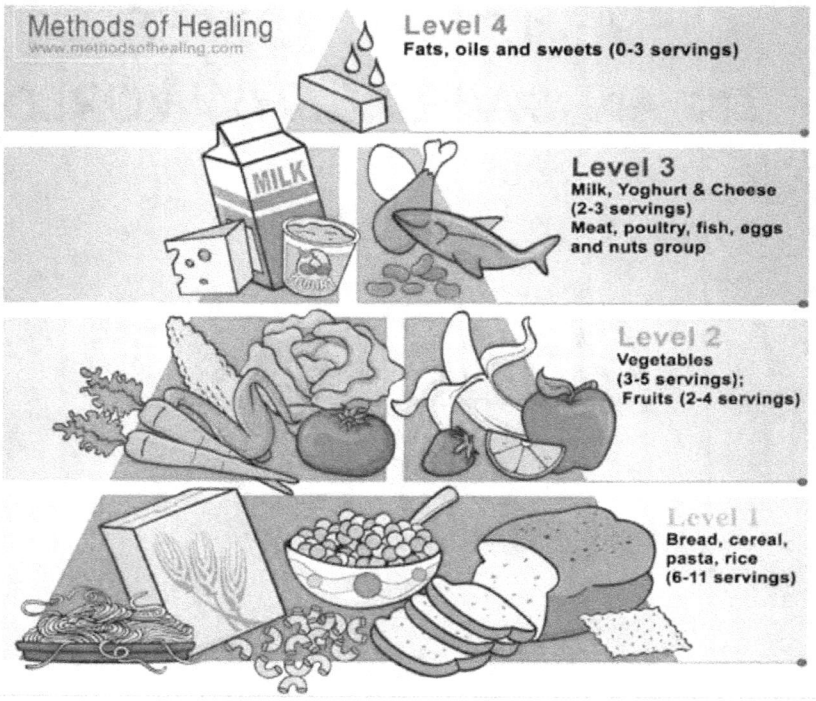

On a daily basis, our bodies are bombarded with all kinds of toxins, germs, and diseases, which can make us very sick. How can we keep healthy? All the natural health gurus tell you, "Just eat right, avoid stress, exercise and take your vitamins." It's very good advice, but for most people it just isn't practical. So, what does the normal person do? That's what this book is designed to help you with.

First of all, let's start with diet. People tell you to eat right, but do you really know what eating right is? For a guideline, we're often given the food pyramid, which is supposed to instill sensible eating habits. They teach it to our children in school. No wonder America is overweight! Let's take a closer look, starting at the bottom.

1. *Bread, cereal, rice, and pasta* - **6-11 servings.** There is a very old saying: "Bread is the staff of life." Until the later part of the nineteenth century, bread basically meant whole grain, ground up - whether wheat, rye, rice, oats, barley, maize, buckwheat or millet. Entire populations lived on whole grain, and little else, and the whole grain was so nutritious and balanced that people were able to get by. Even today, two-thirds of the world is lucky if it can get "bread." If unrefined whole grain is the "bread" you are eating, this part of the pyramid may not be so bad for you, if you can supplement it with some of the other food types.

But nowadays, especially in the United States, "bread" and the other products listed mean *white flour.* It's made up of carbohydrates, which are a form of energy: they convert to glucose or sugar. This sugar can upset the body's blood-sugar balance, and cause fluctuations in energy and mood. You don't want a diet with too many carbohydrates, because the sugar/glucose can make you gain weight; on the other hand, you don't want a diet too *low* in carbohydrates, because it can deplete glycogen, a storage form of glucose stored in the liver and muscles. Without this storage you may run out of energy.

White flour is missing two key constituents, the outside bran layer and the germ (embryo), which are the most nutritious parts of the seed, and are also high in fiber. This can leave you malnourished and constipated.

The more refined foods a person eats, the more insulin the body has to produce to manage it. This leads to rapid weight gain and high triglycerides, which can cause heart disease. The pancreas can become overworked, and you can develop either diabetes (high blood sugar) or hypoglycemia (low blood sugar). Don't be fooled by product labels that say "enriched flour" -- they take out 15 nutrients and add back 4. Something about that just doesn't seem to add up.

Refined flour and sugar also put a strain on our adrenal glands and their ability to produce hormones. There, again, the end result – you put on pounds. Remember, this is how we are told to eat, and America is one of the fattest countries. Gee, wonder why?

2. ***The next group is fruit – 2-4 servings daily.*** Fruits are very healthy for you. They are high in fiber, vitamin C, and natural sugars. Regular consumption of fruit can lower your risk of developing cancer, heart disease, stroke, Alzheimer's disease, and many others.

Fruits that are high in potassium can help to prevent kidney stones, and maybe even prevent bone loss as we age. Fruits are also low-calorie, but can satisfy a craving for "something sweet." When we think of fruit, we normally think of apples, bananas, grapes and such, but we need to remember some vegetables are really fruits, too, such as squash, pumpkin, cucumber, tomatoes, peas, beans, corn, eggplant, and sweet pepper. Don't forget to add these important "fruits" to your diet.

I think, with the wide variety, we need much more than 2-4 servings daily. What do you think?

3. ***Now we come to the vegetables-- 2-3 servings daily.*** Mom really knew what she was talking about when she would tell you to "eat your vegetables" -- this is probably the most important food group.

Dark-green, leafy vegetables are high in iron and calcium, and are great for building strong bones. All vegetables contain vitamins, minerals, fiber and carbohydrates. Eating a diet rich in fruits and vegetables can lower your risk of heart disease and diabetes, as well as protecting you from cancer.

The cruciferous vegetables, such as broccoli and cabbage (to name a couple), have potent anti-cancer properties, but can slow the production of the thyroid hormone. It's best to eat *any* vegetable raw, but especially broccoli.

Go for color – dark green, yellow, red and orange, and eat vegetables daily, with each meal. You can't go wrong on the nutritional value, and you can look for lower blood pressure, less risk of heart disease, cancer, stroke, eye, and digestive problems.

4. *Meat, poultry and eggs - 2-3 servings.* This is the protein category. Your body needs protein to maintain its balance. Fish is included in this category as well, and salmon, trout and herring are rich in omega 3 fatty acids. Processed meats are something you should never eat. When you do eat meat, you need to choose the low-fat or leaner cuts. Meat supplies B-vitamins, and helps you to build healthy blood. If you are a vegetarian, you will need to supplement these in some way.

Eggs have a bad reputation from the American Medical Association, but they are the perfect protein. The yolks do contain cholesterol, but when you look at the overall nutrition of an egg, the good definitely outweighs the bad.

Eggs supply all the essential amino acids, lots of vitamins and minerals and are low in fat. Besides that, they taste good. Who could ask for more?

By the way, your brain is 80% cholesterol – cut it too low and you lose brain function. Cholesterol is also an integral part of your body's repair mechanism for damaged arterial walls.

Our bodies need cholesterol - listen to your doctor and get your numbers below 200, and see what happens to your brain function and arteries! But that's another story.

5. *Milk, yogurt and cheese - 2-3 servings.* Humans are the only mammal to continue to drink milk on a regular basis after being weaned. One thing to remember: milk was designed to allow a baby calf to at least triple its weight in the first year of life. Dairy products cause mucus, which can make asthma or any breathing problem worse. And they are very constipating; this can lead to colon cancer. Aged cheese can cause migraines.

Okay, I know a lot of you won't agree with me on those statements, and milk does have nutritional value. (How else could a cow be so healthy?) These are just some ideas for you to think about.

If you are going to drink milk, you need to find someone with a cow and get fresh milk. It tastes completely different from what you buy at the store, and is much better. What comes from the store is from cows that are pumped full of hormones, antibiotics (and who knows what else?), and we give this to our children. At least, get fresh milk with no additives.

6. **And the last category – fats, oils and sweets – use sparingly.** Not much I can add to that. However, never use any type of oil except cold-pressed extra virgin olive oil. Canola oil should only be used as a lubricant, not taken internally. It can cause cancer and all kinds of diseases. Don't even ask about vegetable oil!

Margarine is another one of my pet peeves -- it's just one molecule away from plastic. Margarine was designed to fatten turkeys. When the turkeys all died, they decided to market it and sell it to us. It's not really a food, and has no nutritional value whatsoever. Try leaving it on the counter for a few days, and see what happens -- no bugs, no mold, nothing. It will sit there – just melted plastic.

Pure butter is so much healthier for you. As a matter of fact, eating butter actually increases the absorption of nutrients from other foods. It is no contest in the battle of butter vs. margarine!

Well, you now have my opinion of the food pyramid. But it's being taught to our children at a very young age. They grow up thinking they should be eating this way, and this is what contributes to our overweight society.

I would re-work it as follows:

Vegetables, 6-11 servings

Fruits, 3-4 servings

Meat, poultry and eggs, 2-3 servings

Bread, pasta, cereal, rice, 1-2 servings and then
   ONLY whole grains

Fats, oils and sweets – sparingly.

If we all ate this way, you would see a huge turnaround in health, weight loss and general well-being.

Dr. Miles' Food pyramid

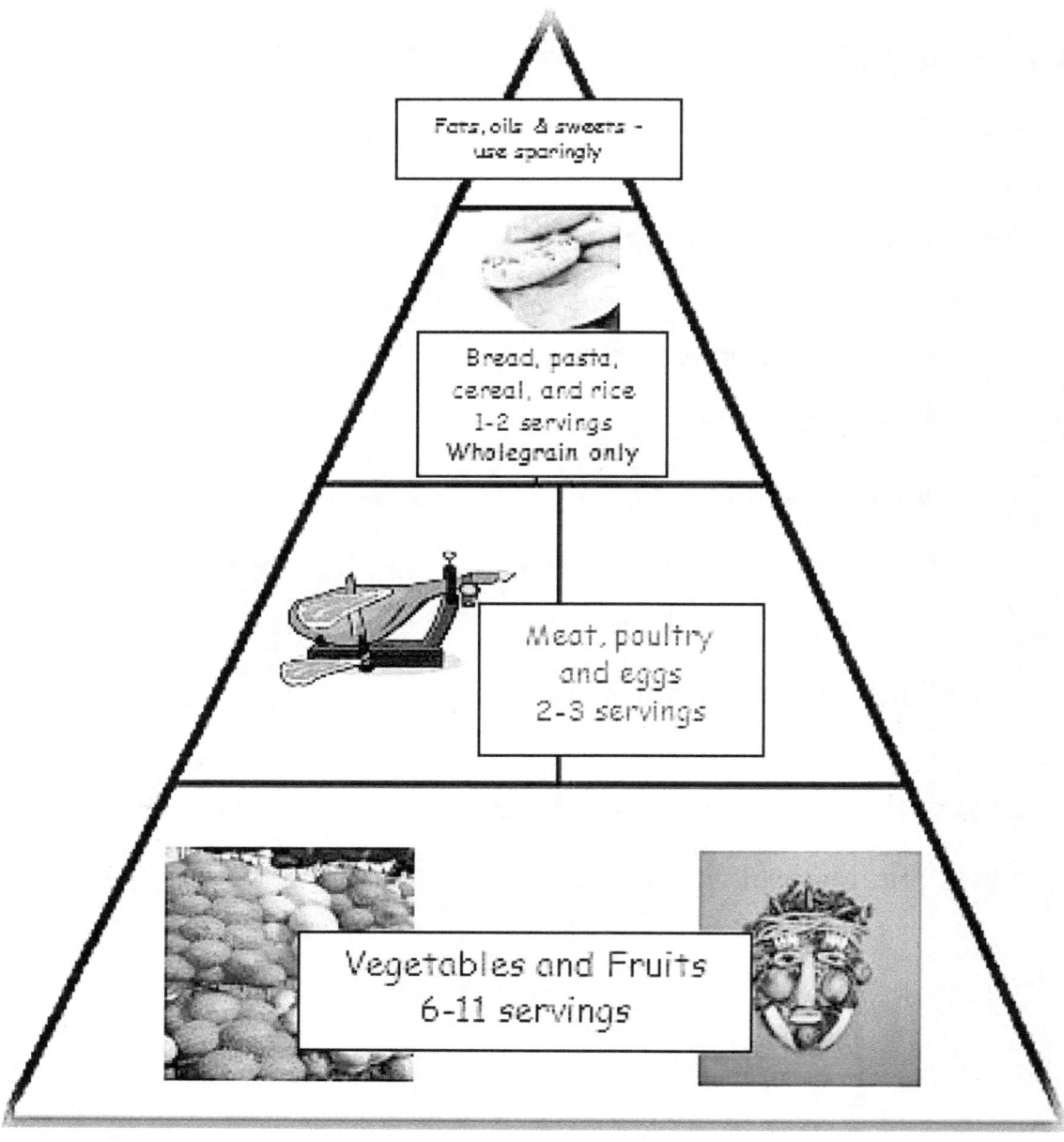

Fats, oils & sweets - use sparingly

Bread, pasta, cereal, and rice 1-2 servings Wholegrain only

Meat, poultry and eggs 2-3 servings

Vegetables and Fruits 6-11 servings

HEALTHY CHOICES
IN AN *UNHEALTHY* WORLD

CHAPTER 2.
REDUCING STRESS

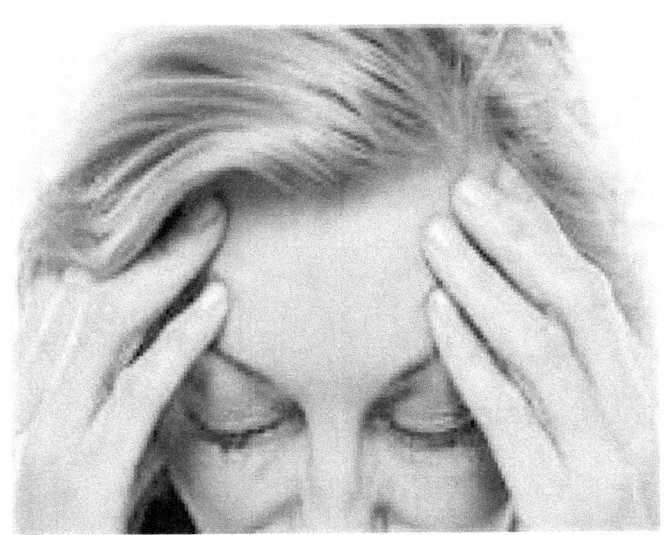

STRESS

Stress! We're always hearing about stress, but just what is it?

It can be a killer. It often goes unnoticed, but leads to stroke, and is a more dangerous risk factor for heart attack and cancer than cigarette smoking and high cholesterol. Every week 95 million Americans take medication to control it.

We all need to get a handle on whatever is causing our stressful situations. When you are under stress, you may suffer some of the following symptoms:

1. Your heart will speed up;

2. The tension in your muscles increases;

3. Digestion stops or really slows because you need energy elsewhere;

4. Your breathing speeds up because you need more oxygen to the muscles;

5. The blood flow to your brain and muscles increases 400 percent, taking blood away from the rest of the body.

Sometimes this is good -- we need this *rush* in an emergency. I'm sure we've all heard stories of someone having the strength to lift a car when a loved one was trapped underneath. If we need to lift a car, this is great, but on a daily basis it will wear out our bodies. It exhausts the adrenal glands, causing them to slow down or quit their production of hormones; they just basically burn out. That is where vitamins become very important, but we'll get to that later.

Just a few of the consequences of stress are:

1. Increase in blood pressure – increasing your risk for heart attack and stroke;

2. Headaches, back pain, chronic fatigue, digestive problems;

3. Decrease in the power of your immune system, which makes you more likely to catch colds and other illnesses;

4. Diminished sexual desire;

5. Worsening asthma;

6. Behaviors that cause body-stress, such as drinking alcohol, using drugs, cigarette smoking and overeating. And stress also makes it very hard to give them up, and have improved health.

7. Weight gain. When our adrenals and thyroid burn out due to chronic stress, our hormone production slows or stops, and we gain weight. This weight becomes very difficult to lose.

Our world is very stressful. Kids, jobs, taking care of a home, money worries -- you name it, we are faced with it on a daily basis. Ideally, we should take time each day to meditate and/or pray. Our spiritual connection with God will strengthen us and give us someone to turn to in our times of trouble. With our busy schedules, it isn't always possible to set aside times for this, so where does that leave us? There are still options for coping with stress, and that is what this chapter is all about.

We have to deal with three kinds of stress – situational, body and emotional, and you use different approaches for them. Let's take a deeper look at each type.

Situational Stress

This type of stress can occur anywhere. Anytime you can't work your way out of an unpleasant situation, you encounter situational stress. Home, office, school, driving, and social activities – all of these can result in situational stress. To better deal with them, you have to break it down and size it up. It's like the old saying, "How do you eat an elephant? -- One bite at a time."

1. Look at the size of the problem – is it too big for you to handle? Is it really an elephant, or does it just seem that way at this moment? How much control do you really have over the situation?

2. Take charge, and gain as much control as possible. It may not be much, but do what you can.

3. Gather information about the situation. The more you have, the better you can deal with it. For instance, if there has been an accident, make sure everyone is safe and getting the attention they need.

4. Don't feel like you are the only one who can solve the problem. There may be other people to lend a hand -- friends and/or family, people in your community. Ask someone to help. No matter what has happened, you are not alone.

5. Your reaction is always the one thing you can control. No matter what is happening, *you* are in control of your reactions and emotions. It may be the <u>only</u> thing you can control, so control it.

6. If you are caught in an ongoing situation, and can't regain control, you might consider short-term therapy. Sometimes another person's objective point of view can really shine a new light on a problem -- maybe turn your elephant into a mouse!

Emotional Stress

Emotional stress is often self-created. It begins as a traumatic event in a person's life that causes severe strain on the nervous system. This could be a death in the family, divorce, loss of a job, birth of a child, life-threatening illness, or anything of this nature. Emotional stress is not sudden, but is brought on by unresolved stress. As emotional stress increases, the problem recreates itself, and causes more stress -- a vicious cycle. You have the feeling that you just can't come to terms with this event. You can't think your way out. This unresolved stress leads to anger, anxiety and depression.

Anger - this emotion can come from a feeling of helplessness because you cannot change the issue. You cannot gain control and therefore feel helpless.

Anxiety – This emotion occurs when you want to do something one way and it turns out another. For instance, you are a public speaker and you want to give a polished presentation, but it turns out all wrong -- you say the wrong things, your equipment fails, and everything goes badly.

Or maybe you're preparing a large meal for family and friends, and the main course burns. These are some of the things that cause anxiety.

Depression – This emotion is usually last on the scale, and the most extreme. Depression is a feeling that all is lost – you will never regain control and you have completely given up hope. At this time, most of all, you need your positive mind-set to take over, but it's almost impossible for this to happen. When the stress continues and you can't think yourself out, then the anger, anxiety and depression just get worse. You must find a way to break the cycle. What it all boils down to is, you must pull yourself out. Remember, the one thing you can control in a stressful situation is your reaction. Depending on your reaction, you can make a situation either more stressful or less.

Emotional stress can affect you in many ways. Did you ever notice that you make it through a very trying time just fine, only to be hit afterwards with a migraine, the flu, or an injury? These are signs of emotional stress -- your system is overloaded, and has to have a release. When you're worried and stressed, your immune system can't work properly, and you are more susceptible to illness. Next time you have a nagging headache, brain fog, forgetfulness or any unexplained symptom, think about your stress level. These symptoms are not always due to an illness -- they <u>can</u> simply be stress.

Body Stress

This kind of stress will cause physical symptoms. Examples are abuse to the body, such as drugs, alcohol, cigarettes, or neglect, from lack of sleep or not getting proper nutrition. Situational and Emotional stress usually always lead to body stress. Some of the symptoms may include overeating, under-eating, withdrawing from social activities, crying spells, conflicts, and as already mentioned, drugs and alcohol abuse. Body stress can make you age faster by causing changes in the immune system that hinder the brain from blocking certain toxins and other harmful substances. Prolonged stress places strain on your brain, which can cause conditions such as functional decline, cardiovascular disease and even some cancers.

MANAGING STRESS

What can I do? You've been under prolonged stress, and need to make changes. Where do you start?

1. **First of all, identify the cause.** Is it a death, divorce, job, whatever – just give it a name. Think back to when the worst part of the stress started, and pinpoint it.

2. **Now analyze the situation.** Is there really anything you can do to control the circumstances? Often, the only thing we can control is our reaction. Change your focus, but don't try to change everything at once. Focus on one part of the problem that is giving you such trouble, and try to slowly adjust your reaction to that part.

3. **Check out alternative viewpoints.** Sometimes an objective person can turn you completely around.

4. **Get away from the problem.** Go on a vacation, or if that's not practical, go shopping – get out for the day. At least try to get away a few minutes each day. Take some time for yourself. Be selfish. You need to heal and regroup. You are important.

   Go easy on yourself. Don't let the small stuff get to you. Just do the really important things, and let the small stuff wait. Maybe you just can't face another load of laundry – so let it wait until tomorrow. Go take a walk.

5. **Do something for others.** Try one random act of kindness each day. It will return to you at least threefold. Doing for others will take your mind off your problems and yourself. Don't bury yourself in self-pity. No matter how bad you think it is, you can always find someone with worse problems than you.

   Get plenty of sleep. If you wake up in the night, and your problems hit you, try telling yourself that now is not the time to think about them, it is time for sleep. Lack of rest will only aggravate stress. Try to relax and sleep. Each time a bad thought comes into your head, push it out. If you can't push it out, read, watch TV, or do anything necessary to distract yourself. Don't let your thoughts control you!

6. **Learn to relax.** Prayer and meditation are wonderful. For me, when I quiet the mind, I believe I connect with God, who brings peace, love and stillness. I recently lost my grandmother, which has affected me deeply. Whenever I get her on my mind and am missing her, I know all I have to do is "phone home." God is always waiting with a comforting hand to soothe and bring me peace. It is the same for any problem -- prayer and meditation will cure whatever ails me!

   Work – physical activity is a great stress reliever. Ideally, you should walk at least 10,000 steps a day (roughly 5 miles). Get a pedometer and measure the distance you walk. If it's cold outside, get a treadmill. Any kind of movement is good. Put on a perky song and dance!!

7. **Try to be positive.** Listen to your internal dialogue. Are you telling yourself how horrible it is, or how well you can cope? Are you getting stuck on the small stuff, and not seeing the forest for the trees? Look at the beauty around you. Make a list of all the good things in your life -- ignore the bad. Sit down and actually <u>do</u> this -- I bet you'll be surprised just how many good things you really have. Smile at everyone you meet. You never know what a difference it might make in someone's day.

8. **Watch a funny movie – listen to upbeat songs.** So many studies have been made on laughter. Some people have cured cancer with it, and laughter will relax the entire body.

We always get a laugh out of my son and grandson -- every time they start really laughing they take the hiccups. It's just so funny watching them try to laugh and hiccup at the same time! Laughter also supports the immune system and releases endorphins, the feel-good chemicals of the body that can give you a very good feeling, and temporary relieve pain. A good belly laugh can relieve tension and stress, help the blood vessels and improve heart function. Humor can change your perspective, make situations feel less threatening, and help you see things in a different light.

Laughing with others is even more powerful than laughing alone. It strengthens relationships and heals resentments. I believe we were meant to be happy. A baby smiles during the first few weeks of life (it's not gas), and laughs out loud at a few months old. Think how precious it is to hear that baby laugh. Think of happy moments in your life. Spend more time with happy people. Laughter is very contagious.

WORRY

I have just finished a long section on stress, without mentioning worry. But the two go hand-in-hand. Usually people who are "stressed-out" are intense worriers.

I come from a long line of worriers, but am determined to break the cycle. My great-grandmother used to tell of a woman who never married and lived alone. One day some neighbors came to visit and found her crying. They asked what was wrong and she told them she was thinking about how horrible it would have been if she had married, had a child and an anvil fell on its head and killed it. I think that is worry to the extreme! My mother's family has all been this way. They worry over the least little thing. How does it stop? I know my family is not the only one with the problem, so I decided to add this chapter.

Some worry is good. It may make you take action and solve a problem. But most worry becomes a problem all of itself. You can lose all your emotional energy and motivation. None of these "what ifs" are productive. You feel like a nervous wreck – no sleep, edgy all day, snappy with friends and family, headaches and body aches from all the tension in the muscles.

What makes someone a chronic worrier? Let's start at the beginning – life is uncertain. Uncertainty is something chronic worriers cannot accept -- they need to know *exactly* how something is going to turn out. By focusing on all the bad things that might happen, you miss the good things that are already happening. Focus on the positive. "Every cloud has a silver lining." -- I know that is an old statement, but it's true. There is always good around you, you just don't choose to see it sometimes. Life is uncertain, it changes every day, and we can't predict what will happen. We just have to let it play out. Sometimes when I am trying to make a decision and the answer just won't come, I just let it play out. I stay focused on the positive, and usually it turns out better than I expected.

Create a "worry time." Set aside a small amount of time each day to worry. Do this early in the day -- maybe 1:00 p.m. to 1:20 p.m. If you do it later, it could keep you awake at night if you haven't resolved everything.

Only worry during this time of the day. If you think of something outside of your "worry time," tell yourself that you can't worry now, but that you will at your official time. Put it on a list and review your list during your "worry time."

Get rid of the negative thoughts. Challenge them – what would you say to your best friend if he/she had this worry? Play them out in your mind, and identify the problem. Ask yourself why you think this is true. Is there a better way to look at the situation? How is this worry going to help me? How is it going to hurt me? Will it really change the situation? Can I control the situation? If it is a situation you cannot control, worry won't change it. All the worry in the world never changed any situation, but just made the worrier miserable. Worry is like a rocking chair, it keeps you busy, but you don't get anywhere. The "managing stress" section of this book also applies here. You need to relax and take care of yourself. Don't worry, be happy!

HEALTHY CHOICES
IN AN *UNHEALTHY* WORLD

CHAPTER 3
EXERCISE

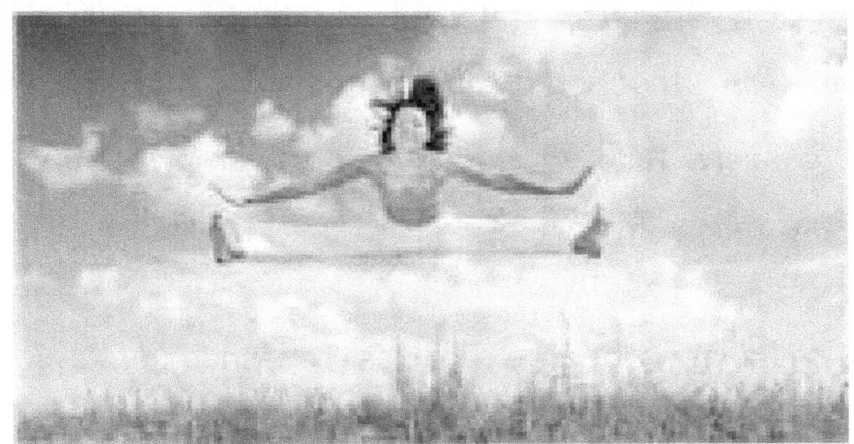

EXERCISE

This will probably be the shortest chapter in this book. Everyone knows the benefits of exercise, so I'm not going to spend much time here. All exercise is good. As we age, our bodies start to lose muscle mass. Exercise prevents this, and enhances our physical appearance and well-being. It strengthens our muscles and keeps us healthy. Everyone can benefit from exercise -- you are never too young or too old.

There are all kinds of exercise videos to try, if you are motivated enough to put one in the DVD and work-out by yourself.

There are also exercise centers, which offer membership. Some of these work on structured circuit training, and target the entire body. Some centers turn you loose to do your own thing -- whatever works best for you.

One of the very best exercises for anybody is just plain, old walking. Shoot for a target of 10,000 steps a day, roughly 5 miles. If you're not up to doing 5 miles, do 3, or even half a mile -- anything is better than none. Start small, and gradually increase it. You'll soon notice a big difference in the way you move and the way you feel.

Exercise can be a treatment for disease. High blood pressure, heart problems, diabetes, arthritis, insomnia, depression, and obesity are just a few that can see tremendous gains from exercise. It also strengthens our immune system and brain function.

Most people stop exercising because of a lack of motivation. If this is your problem, do simple things. Take the stairs instead of the elevator, park further from your destination, for a few extra steps. Get a dog – they love to take walks. Studies show that dog owners walk twice as much as non-dog owners. Exercise with a friend, or form a walking club. Just move!!!!!

Always remember to drink plenty of water before, during and after exercise. Do warm-up stretches for about 5-10 minutes to help the muscles. Remember, you shouldn't eat a big meal closer than 2 hours prior to or after intense exercise. Most of all, listen to your body, and, if it's too much, stop. You are working on improving your health, not making it worse.

HEALTHY CHOICES

IN AN *UNHEALTHY* WORLD

CHAPTER 4

NUTRITION

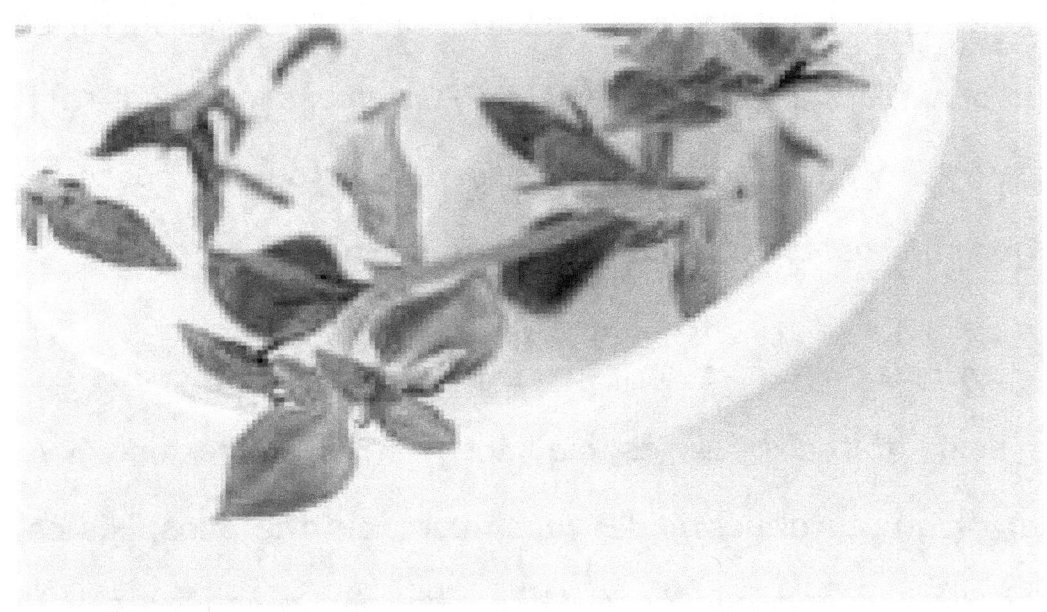

NUTRITION

Proper nutrition is essential for good health. Years ago, you could depend on your food for your nutrition, but that is not the case now. Soils have been depleted, and food is picked green or grown in a greenhouse.

We also import a lot of our food. Go into any grocery store, and look at the labels. You'll find very few that are a product of the United States. I was going to buy a cantaloupe at the grocery, and found that most came from Mexico or somewhere else outside the United States.

Our area is full of local growers. These people need the business and have really good produce, but the grocery owners still choose to import our food. I wouldn't buy my cantaloupe or produce from the grocery -- I went to the local growers. If you are concerned about nutrition and taste, I suggest you do the same.

Pesticides are also an issue. I know a man who grows cabbage to sell to some of the groceries in a nearby city. He uses only a very small amount of a natural pesticide, which controls the bugs. His cabbage is huge, beautiful and bug free. When he was ready to sell it to the grocery he was told that he had to dip it in a strong pesticide.

Mind you, it had no bugs, but they would not buy it until he treated it. Pesticides do not completely wash off with water, and we ingest them.

I think it is a conspiracy for population control. If it will kill a bug, it will kill you!

When shopping for food, the best places in the grocery are around the perimeter, where all the produce and fresh vegetables are located. Even though you have to watch out for the pesticides, they're still the healthiest items in the store.

To get the most nutrition out of your food, you need to eat it as close to raw as possible. If you must cook it, just lightly steam it, to preserve as much of the nutrients as possible. For cooking, use pots and pans made of cast iron, glass or stainless steel. Whatever you do, don't cook with aluminum, which is absorbed into food, and can cause many health problems. High acid foods, especially, pull out more aluminum than anything else -- you can even *taste* it. If you can afford it, throw the aluminum away -- don't even feed the dog out of it.

Teflon is another thing to throw out. The following is a quote from an Associated Press article published in 2005:

"A controversial chemical used by DuPont Co. to make the nonstick substance Teflon poses more of a <u>cancer risk</u> than indicated in a draft assessment by the Environmental Protection Agency, an independent review board has found.

"The EPA stated earlier this year that its draft risk assessment of perfluorooctanoic acid and its salts found "suggestive evidence" of potential human carcinogenicity, based on animal studies.

"In a draft report released Monday, the majority of members on an EPA scientific advisory board that reviewed the agency's report concluded that PFOA, also known as C-8, is "likely" to be carcinogenic to humans, and that the EPA should conduct cancer risk assessments for a variety of <u>tumors</u> found in mice and rats.

"Environmentalists hailed the report, which will be discussed by EPA officials and SAB members in a public teleconference July 6, as an important step in holding government regulators and the Delaware-based chemical giant accountable.

"The board's findings will increase pressure on the EPA to conduct human <u>health</u> risk assessments for liver, breast, pancreatic and testicular cancer, as well as PFOA's potentially toxic effects on the immune system, said Richard Wiles, senior vice president for the Environmental Working Group, an advocacy and research organization.

"'This is contrary to the recommendation of the EPA staff and is a very important conclusion,' said Wiles, adding that it would be very unlikely for the board to make any significant changes before issuing its final report for review by the EPA.

"'This makes it hard for the EPA not to move forward aggressively,' he said."

This was published in 2005, 6 years ago. I don't know about you, but I haven't seen the EPA move forward aggressively.

You also need to be particular with the microwave. Never cook anything in plastic. Once again, use only glass. This way you don't have to be concerned if your plastic is microwave safe or not. Some sources say it is okay and others say it is not. Better to be safe than sorry, so use only glass.

HEALTHY CHOICES
IN AN *UNHEALTHY* WORLD

CHAPTER 5
VITAMINS

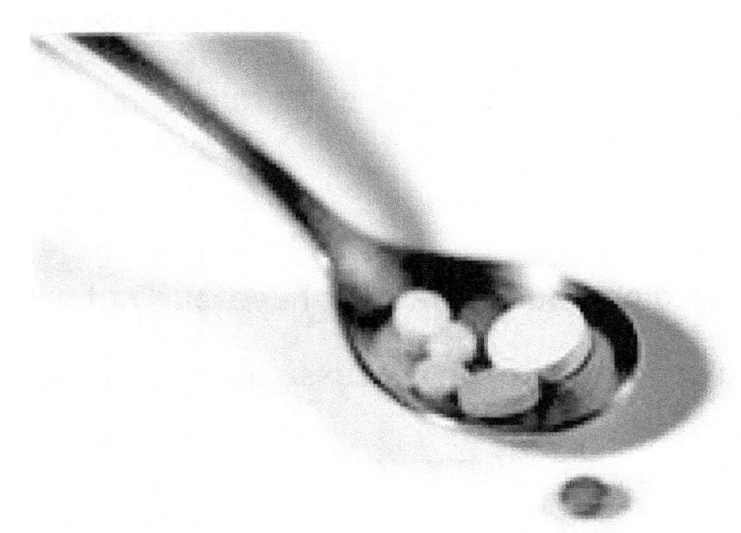

VITAMINS

Vitamins are essential to human growth. They build a strong body. As the fetus begins to develop in the womb, it needs certain nutrients at certain times. These nutrients have to be present to develop skin, muscle and bone, and if they're not available at the precise time, a deficiency can develop, causing permanent damage.

After we are born, nutrients are just as important. If a child lacks the necessary amount of iron by age 2, the brain won't develop properly, and the damage will be permanent.

As we continue to grow, we need a steady flow of vitamins and minerals for proper development, just like the fetus. As we enter into each stage of development we require certain amounts of vitamins and minerals to complete growth.

After we become adults, we still need our nutrients to maintain cells, tissues and organs, and for processing carbohydrates, protein and fats. Nutrients give us energy and optimal brain function.

_____

There are 13 vitamins, divided into two kinds: fat-soluble and water-soluble. The four fat-soluble vitamins (A, D, E, and K) are stored in the body. They can accumulate, and you can overdose on them, but a deficiency is generally more of a concern than an overdose.

The 9 water-soluble vitamins (8 B-vitamins and vitamin C) are excreted from the body, if not used. They need to be consumed on a daily basis.

Deficiencies can be classified as primary or secondary. A primary deficiency can occur when you don't get enough vitamins from your food or other sources, such as a multivitamin.

A secondary deficiency occurs when something prevents or severely limits your absorption of that vitamin, like excessive alcohol use, cigarette-smoking or medications that deplete the vitamin. Restrictive diets can also be a culprit. Secondary deficiencies are usually lifestyle-related.

Avitaminosis is a catch-all term for any disease caused by long-term vitamin deficiency or a problem with metabolic conversion. The letter of the vitamin in question is added at the end -- for example, *avitaminosis A*.

Some of the diseases caused by vitamin deficiency are:

- night blindness (vitamin A)

- beriberi (thiamine)

- pellagra (niacin)

- megaloblastic anemia (B12)

- scurvy (vitamin C)

- rickets (vitamin D)

- impaired coagulation (vitamin K).

Hypervitaminosis is the term for an overdose of a vitamin. It is also designated by the letter of the vitamin -- for example, *hypervitaminosis A*. High storage levels of any vitamin usually result from taking mega doses of supplements, rather than from food. This occurs more often with the fat-soluble vitamins. Since they are stored in the liver and fatty tissues, they can build up and remain in the body longer than water-soluble vitamins. High doses of minerals can also build up in the body, and cause toxicity and various side effects.

Vitamin-poisoning death is typically uncommon in the United States, as reported by http://www.orthomolecular.org/resources/omns/v05n04.shtml .

"For example, in the United States, overdose exposure to all formulations of 'vitamins' was reported by 62,562 individuals in 2004 (nearly 80% of these exposures were in children under the age of 6), leading to 53 "major" life-threatening outcomes and 2 deaths."

Deficiency in a vitamin is much more of a concern.

But remember, vitamin supplements for children should never be stored in a place accessible to the child. The vitamins taste very good, and if children were to consume the entire bottle, it could be fatal.

NATURAL OR SYNTHETIC

What's the difference?

Synthetic vitamins are manufactured in a laboratory from coal-tar derivatives. They are much cheaper to produce, and therefore the company can make much more profit from them.

Natural vitamins come from food sources, and some contain nutrients that just can't be produced in a laboratory, like Vitamin E. *D-alpha-tocopherol* is the natural form of vitamin E, and *dl-alpha-tocopherol* is the synthetic form. But your body doesn't recognize the synthetic version, and it is excreted. So you need to be sure to check the label when you purchase this vitamin -- you might be flushing your money down the drain!

Vitamin C is another story. Although I always recommend natural vitamins, the synthetic version often works well, provided it has bioflavonoids added to increase absorption. Vitamin C with rose-hips and Ester-C are best, but make sure you don't give your children the chewable kind - it can damage the enamel of their teeth.

One analogy I found on the Internet (www.nutriteam.com) says it perfectly:

"In the laboratory, chemists can duplicate seawater that is chemically identical to natural seawater, but if you put fish in this synthetic water they will die. Obviously, there is a life-supporting difference between natural and synthetic."

Make sure you research your supplements well. Manufacturers can claim a vitamin is "natural" when it contains only 10% natural ingredients. The only way to tell if it is truly natural is to read the label and look for food sources, not chemicals.

"100% organic" is misleading, as well. A molecule only has to have one carbon atom to be certified 100% organic, and these can include coal tar and wood pulp, neither of which you want to consume.

To help you in label reading, this is a chart from the website, www.nutriteam.com. Remember this the next time you're shopping for vitamins.

How to Read Labels

Item:	If source Given Is:	It Is:
Vitamin A	Fish Oils Lemon Grass Acetate Palmitate If source not given	Natural Co-Natural Synthetic Synthetic Synthetic
Vitamin B-Complex	Brewer's Yeast If source not given	Natural Synthetic
Vitamin B1 (Thiamine)	Yeast Thiamine Mononitrate Thiamine Hydrochloride	Natural Synthetic Synthetic
Vitamin B2 (Riboflavin)	Yeast Riboflavin	Natural Synthetic
Pantothenic Acid	Yeast, Rice Bran or Liver Calcium D-Pantothenate	Natural Synthetic
Vitamin B6 (Pyridoxine)	Yeast Pyridoxine Hydrochloride	Natural Synthetic
Vitamin B12	Liver Micro-organism fermentation Cobalamin Concentrate	Natural Co-Natural Co-Natural
PABA	Yeast - Para-aminobenzoic Acid Aminobenzoic Acid	Natural Synthetic
Folic Acid	Yeast or Liver Pteroylglutamic Acid	Natural Synthetic
Inositol	Soy Beans Reduced from Corn	Natural Co-Natural

Choline	Soy Beans Choline Chloride Choline Bitartrate	Natural Synthetic Synthetic
Biotin	Liver d-Biotin	Natural Synthetic
Niacin	Yeast Niacinamide Niacin	Natural Co-Natural Synthetic
Vitamin C (Ascorbic Acid)	Citrus, Rose Hips, Acerola Berries Ascorbic Acid If source not given	Natural Synthetic Synthetic
Vitamin D	Fish Oils Irradiated Ergosteral (Yeast) Calciferol	Natural Synthetic Synthetic
Vitamin E	Veg. Oil, Wheat Germ Oil, or Mixed Tocopherols d-alpha tocopherol * dl-alpha tocopherol	Natural Natural Synthetic
Vitamin F	Essential Fatty Acids	Natural
Vitamin K	Alfalfa Menadione	Natural Synthetic

* The "dl" form of any supplement is synthetic.

INDIVIDUAL VITAMINS

In this section, we'll take the vitamins one by one and study their values.

VITAMIN A

Vitamin A is a fat-soluble vitamin, sometimes called the "miracle" vitamin. Actually, it's a mixture of vitamins, parts of which are stored in the body. Two of the parts are *retinol* and *carotene*. Retinol is found in animal foods, and carotene in plant food.

Sources of Vitamin A include liver, eggs, dairy foods, kidneys, carrots, sweet potatoes, pumpkin, and kale, just to name a few, but it's found in many of our foods. You can often tell just by looking -- the orange foods are high in beta-carotene. The body converts beta-carotene to Vitamin A as needed, and it's not toxic like vitamin A -- what isn't used will be eliminated from the body. It's also an anti-oxidant, and will help protect us from certain forms of cancer and other diseases. Most multivitamins contain a mixture of vitamin A and beta-carotene.

BENEFITS OF VITAMIN A

Some of the benefits of Vitamin A include:

1. Vision – vitamin A is used in the retina of the eye. It allows our eyes to adjust when we come in from light to dark, and allows us to see colors. It helps people with glaucoma, and puts that sparkle back in dry and dull eyes!

2. Anti-oxidant and immune builder – helps to protect us from cancer and other diseases, such as heart disease, stroke, and infections of all kinds - bacterial, parasitic and viral. Helps lower cholesterol. It is essential for children who have poor growth.

3. Strong bones - essential in the formation of strong bones and teeth.

4. Skin - Vitamin A is required for development and maintenance of epithelial cells in the mucous membranes and your skin.

DEFICIENCY OF VITAMIN A

Vitamin A is the most prevalent vitamin deficiency in the world. One of the first symptoms is night blindness. Dryness of the conjunctiva and cornea are problems associated with this important vitamin. Eyes that are dry, itchy and tire easily are usually a warning of not enough Vitamin A. If this deficiency is not corrected, the cornea can ulcerate and you can become permanently blind.

Other symptoms of a deficiency may include loss of the ability to fight infections, dry skin and hair, poor growth, sinusitis, acne, insomnia, fatigue and reproductive difficulties. If you are also deficient in protein, your hair and scalp can become very dry.

VITAMIN A WORKS BEST WITH …

Ideally, you don't want to just take one vitamin. They work best in combinations. When you take vitamin A, you need to include a B-complex, Vitamins C, D and E, essential fatty acids, and choline. To get the very best benefits, add calcium, zinc and phosphorus.

Your need for this vitamin may be increased if you consume alcohol regularly, if you're on a low-fat diet, or you eat a diet high in polyunsaturated fatty acids and smoke. Diabetics and people with underactive thyroid glands typically need more Vitamin A.

Dosage Chart – Office of Dietary Supplements
National Institutes of Health

Recommended Dietary Allowances (RDAs) for vitamin A

Age (years)	Children (mcg RAE)	Males (mcg RAE)	Females (mcg RAE)	Pregnancy (mcg RAE)	Lactation (mcg RAE)
1-3	300 (1,000 IU)				
4-8	400 (1,320 IU)				
9-13	600 (2,000 IU)				
14-18		900 (3,000 IU)	700 (2,310 IU)	750 (2,500 IU)	1,200 (4,000 IU)
19+		900 (3,000 IU)	700 (2,310 IU)	770 (2,565 IU)	1,300 (4,300 IU)

Keep in mind that Vitamin A, taken in large dosages, can be toxic, as it builds up in our bodies. Most healthy adults have a reserve of this vitamin. If you are going to supplement, the safest form is beta-carotene. Beta-carotene is converted to vitamin A as we need it. It is very safe and the only side effect of too much beta-carotene is a yellow tint to the skin, but this poses no health problems.

B-COMPLEX

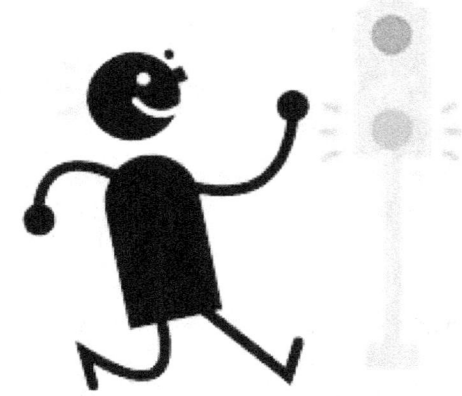

B-complex is a combination of all the water-soluble vitamins (except C). These include B1 (*thiamine*), B2 (*riboflavin*), B3 (*niacin*), B5 (*pantothenic acid*), B6 (*pyridoxine*), B7 (*biotin*), B9 (*folic acid*), and B12 (*cobalamins*).

At one time Vitamin B was thought to be a single nutrient, but researchers discovered later that they consisted of several vitamins. These were given numbers to distinguish them, thus B1, B2, B3 and so on. Other substances in the B-complex family have been discovered, such as *choline, para-aminobenzoic acid* (PABA) and *inositol*. Each member of the B family is needed for a specific function in the human body: B1, B2, B3 and biotin are used in energy production; B6 is needed to metabolize amino acids; and B12 and folic acid work in cell-division.

Since they are water-soluble, they must be replenished on a regular basis, either through food or supplements. What we don't use, we simply excrete in our urine. B-vitamins will color your urine a bright yellow, and many people have said they seem to be flushing money down the drain, but your kidneys use this vitamin as it passes through them, making them work more efficiently.

Sources of B vitamins include whole unprocessed foods, and turkey and tuna are good meat sources. Your diet should include whole grains, potatoes, bananas, beans, and molasses, as these are very good sources for B-vitamins.

B1 - THIAMINE

Thiamine – the first of the B-vitamins, was isolated in the 1930s. It helps the body convert carbohydrates into energy -- in other words, it breaks down sugars in the diet. Every cell in the body depends on this vitamin for fuel. It is also needed for the heart, muscles and nervous system.

DEFICIENCY OF B1

A deficiency of this vitamin is rare, but people who consume alcohol regularly, have liver or kidney problems, or eat a lot of sweets, soft drinks and processed foods can be at risk. Deficiency symptoms include loss of appetite, poor digestion, insomnia, slow heartbeat, irritability, and digestive disorders. If this continues, it can develop into beriberi, which is a condition involving a rapid heartbeat, confusion, muscle-wasting and nerve problems. It is very rarely seen in the United States. Generally, the only people who have to be concerned about a deficiency are chronic alcoholics.

SOURCES

Good sources include cereals, pasta, whole grains, lean meat, beans, eggs, and most vegetables. The very best sources are brewer's yeast, egg yolks, fish, liver and whole grains. If you eat a diet that is high in carbohydrates, you increase the need for thiamine.

DOSAGE

Your daily needs are based on the amount of calories you consume each day, but as a general guideline, dosages are →**1.1 milligrams for men** and →**0.8 milligrams for women**, every day. Of course, if you are pregnant or lactating, you'll need more. This dosage should be included in a complete B-complex supplement.

B2 - RIBOFLAVIN

Riboflavin, the second vitamin in the B family, was also isolated in the 1930s. Whenever you take a B-complex, you can always tell if it contains riboflavin, because that's the one responsible for turning your urine a fluorescent yellow. This is the only vitamin that colors the urine.

Riboflavin is manufactured in the body by the intestinal flora, and is very easily absorbed. We need it there in our digestive tracts to keep the mucous membranes healthy. There is a constant need for this vitamin, because very little is stored. The body uses it to metabolize amino acids, carbohydrates and fatty acids. It also activates Vitamin B6, which helps the body produce the niacin to boost the adrenal gland. We need it for healthy red blood cells, production of antibodies, and growth. B2 also works to relive eye-fatigue, and may prevent or treat cataracts.

SOURCES

Eggs, nuts, green leafy vegetables, milk, and lean meats are all good sources of riboflavin.

DEFICIENCY OF B2

Riboflavin is found in so many foods that a deficiency is almost unheard-of, but symptoms would include anemia, skin disorders, sore throat, mouth sores, and swelling of mucous membranes. Since it is water-soluble and the excess leaves your body, there is no known toxicity from this vitamin.

DOSAGE

RDA is →**1.7 mg each day for an adult male** and →**1.3 mg each day for an adult female.**

RIBOFLAVIN AND MIGRAINES

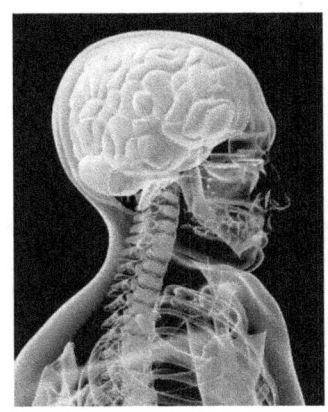

Migraines are caused by inflammation of the blood vessels in the brain. No one knows the exact cause, although many triggers have been noted. Riboflavin, in even a small dose, such as 25 mg a day, has helped in the prevention and treatment of migraines, because it stimulates energy production, and migraine sufferers seem to have low energy production in the brain cells. Add a dose of magnesium, which also works with energy production in the brain, and you just may have found your cure. If you suffer from migraines, this might be worth a try.

B3 - NIACIN

Niacin, the third member of the B family, was discovered in 1867 by Hugo Weidel. There are different members of this family of compounds, but the only two we are going to be concerned with are *niacin* and *niacinamide (or nicotinamide)*. These two are identical in activity, but work a little differently in the body. *Niacin* will reduce cholesterol and triglycerides, and cause flushing, while *niacinamide* does not.

Niacin works with DNA repair, and helps to produce hormones in the adrenal glands. It can also be helpful for people who have heart disease or have had a heart attack.

For over 50 years, doses of niacin have been known to reduce cholesterol. Some doctors prescribe niacin instead of chemical cholesterol-lowering medication, because niacin is much easier on your system than the harsh side effects of the other cholesterol-lowering medications.

Niacin opens the blood vessels and increases blood flow, thus the niacin flush. This flush is not dangerous or harmful in any way -- it is just improved blood-flow. As the blood-flow increases, you'll be getting rid of waste products and cleaning out your capillaries. Sometimes, with the "flush," you'll feel itchy. This is caused from the production of histamine, which is just part of the process.

Niacin can be effective in weight loss, not directly, but by reducing stress and increasing energy. It also aids in digestion and regulates blood pressure, and may alleviate migraine headaches.

Atherosclerosis is another disease that may benefit from niacin. With the "flush," you have better blood flow and the blood vessels relax, which can help prevent that plaque buildup along the blood vessels that causes blockages. Thus, you also prevent heart attacks and strokes.

Niacinamide may be a therapy to prevent sugar diabetes or at least delay the need for insulin.

Osteoarthritis, along with rheumatoid arthritis, can be improved with a dose of niacin. Niacinamide can increase joint mobility and decrease muscle/joint fatigue. It is an anti-inflammatory, and can also increase muscle strength.

DEFICIENCY OF B3

A deficiency is rare in most countries, and is usually found only in areas of poverty, malnutrition or chronic alcoholism. A mild deficiency can slow your metabolism, which can decrease your tolerance to cold temperatures. Irritability, poor concentration, depression, restlessness, anxiety and fatigue are also symptoms of a deficiency. Severe deficiency is known as pellagra.

SOURCES

Niacin is common in a variety of foods, including liver, fish (tuna and salmon), peanuts, chicken, beef, tomatoes, leaf vegetables, sweet potatoes, asparagus, whole grains, and carrots, just to name a few.

DOSAGE OF B3

This is a water-soluble vitamin that doesn't build up in your body, so you must replenish it every day. RDA is →20 mg, but it's usually supplemented at →100 mg. This is the most powerful of the B-vitamins, and the best-known. Make sure you get your daily requirement!

B5 - PANTOTHENIC ACID

This is number 5 in the B-complex family. Once again, this is a water-soluble vitamin, and needs to be replenished on a daily basis. This vitamin breaks-down carbohydrates, proteins and fats for energy.

B5 helps in the secretion of hormones, which supports the adrenal gland. Hormones help the metabolism, help allergies, and provide us with healthy skin, nerves and muscles. I have even heard that it fights wrinkles and keeps our hair from turning gray!

It's important for a healthy digestive tract. With a surplus of this vitamin, you use *other* vitamins more effectively. As with the whole B-complex family, B5 helps to manage stress, whether physical, psychological, stress from migraines, or chronic fatigue syndrome. It can also assist in alcohol or smoking cessation.

SOURCES

Pantothenic acid is found in almost all foods, including cheese, corn, peas, eggs, most meats, kale, broccoli, tomatoes, milk, sweet potatoes, cauliflower, salmon, and peanuts. But heating or canning will destroy it.

B5 DEFICIENCY

A deficiency is virtually nonexistent, since B5 is present in so many foods. But if you *were* deficient, the symptoms would include: fatigue, depression, headaches, tingling in the hands, nausea and cardiac instability. You can also have sleep disturbances, cramps, and muscle weakness, abdominal pains, numbness.

If you are under stress, have a lot of allergies, eat a diet high in refined foods or consume alcohol on a regular basis, you might have a shortage of this vitamin.

DOSAGE

There is no specific established RDA for B5, although →**4-7 mg.** for adults is about normal. There is no known toxicity, though large amounts can cause diarrhea. Like all B vitamins, B5 is best taken in a B-complex formula. The B family works together, and they need each other for the best results.

B6 - PYRIDOXINE

According to Phyllis Balch (<u>Prescription for Nutritional Healing</u>), Vitamin B6 "...is involved in more bodily functions than almost any other single nutrient."

Like other B-vitamins, B6 helps the body convert protein, fat and carbohydrates into energy, keeps our immune and nervous systems healthy, fights heart disease, and regulates hormone production. It can be useful in the treatment of diabetes, heart disease and varicose veins.

B6 is *essential* for cardiovascular and circulatory health. It keeps the red blood cells from clumping together to form clots, which is critical in cardiovascular problems. It also helps in balancing sodium and potassium. Do you know someone who has congestive heart failure? This is the vitamin for them. It has not been proven, but is believed that B6 can help with PMS, builds cancer immunity and may even help with carpal tunnel syndrome.

SOURCES

All foods contain some B6. But especially look for whole grains, bread, liver, bananas, carrots, chicken, eggs, milk, oatmeal, fish, poultry, potatoes, spinach, and green beans. B6 is sensitive to light and heat, so you can lose a lot during the cooking process.

DEFICIENCY OF B6

A deficiency is rare, but if you do develop a deficiency, it's usually associated with poor absorption of nutrients. Deficiency symptoms could include itchy or peeling skin, cracked lips, inflamed mouth and tongue, confusion, insomnia, and poor coordination.

B6 DOSAGE

About →2 mg. daily for an adult is a good dosage. Remember, when I tell you these dosages, these are the Recommended Daily Allowance (RDA), which only means that it is enough to keep you from being *deficient*, not necessarily what you need to be *healthy*. This is another water-soluble vitamin, which means you need to replenish it daily.

B7 - BIOTIN

The "hair and skin vitamin," or, as it is better known, the "beauty vitamin." The word *Biotin* comes from the Greek word *bios*, which means "life." Without this vitamin certain enzymes won't work properly, and complications can occur. Biotin works with the skin, intestinal tract and the nervous system. Without biotin you could develop low blood sugar, high blood ammonia or acidosis. Biotin is also needed to form fatty acids and glucose, essential for producing energy. Like all other B vitamins, it helps metabolize carbohydrates, fats, amino acids and proteins.

Biotin is also called Vitamin H, because of the German words for "hair and skin," which are "*haar und haut.*" This is the vitamin to use if you have hair-loss or brittle fingernails. It is added to many beauty compounds such as shampoo and lotion, but biotin is not absorbed through the skin, and will not work this way. The only way to get it to your hair, skin or nails is to ingest it.

This is often the vitamin that gets left out or added in very small amounts to a B-complex. Big vitamin companies try to put together the cheapest vitamin compound they can, and biotin is relatively expensive, so they cut the amount. Always read the label. If you're not getting enough biotin in your B-complex, buy it separately and supplement it. Watch the price -- if it's too cheap, you're not really getting biotin.

SOURCES

Good sources of Biotin include organ meats, oatmeal, egg yolk, bananas, nuts, dairy products, chocolate, fish, kidneys, molasses, beans, bread and brewer's yeasts. Food-processing techniques, such as canning, freezing, and cooking can destroy biotin. Try to eat your food as near the raw state as possible to get not only more of this vitamin but of all the others as well.

DEFICIENCY

A deficiency is rare, but can be caused by eating a large amount of egg whites (about 20 eggs a day). The egg white contains a protein, avidin, which binds biotin. Symptoms of a biotin deficiency include, hair loss, dry or brittle hair, dry skin, rashes, and fungal infections. If you have a biotin deficiency from eating too many egg whites, a change of diet is in order.

B7 DOSAGE

Typically, a good dose of biotin is about →**300 mcg daily**, an adequate one about →**30-100 mcg** daily. If you need to treat hair or nail problems, you could take up to 2,500 mcg daily. Higher amounts have been used to reduce blood sugar levels in diabetics. No side effects have been noted. As with other B's, biotin works best in a B-complex. It is water-soluble and what you don't use, you lose. It does need to be replenished daily.

B9 - FOLIC ACID

Folic acid is essential for human growth and development, and crucial for proper brain function and cell-duplication. Whenever cell growth is very active, as it is during pregnancy, the demand for B9 increases. This is because B6, B9, and B12 work closely together to help the body use iron properly, by regulating formation of the red blood cells. They also work to eliminate *homocysteine*, which can cause early heart attacks or strokes.

Folic acid can stimulate the production of stomach acid to aid digestion, can help maintain a healthy liver, and will increase the appetite. It can also protect against parasites and food poisoning, and give you prettier, healthier skin as a bonus!

It is vital to make sure you get enough of this vitamin during pregnancy, as it can prevent certain birth defects. Also, it is useful with a condition known as *cervical dysplasia*, an abnormal pap smear. This can often be corrected by supplementing with folic acid, which works with the reproduction of cells. You want to grow healthy cells. If you have this condition, you might try 1,000 mcg daily for 3-4 months. This may improve the cervical cells. Again, since folic acid works with the reproduction of cells, it also works in the treatment of cancer.

Cancer is caused by one cell mutating and others following. If you have enough folic acid, and your cells are reproducing normally, you're less likely to develop cancer.

SOURCES

Folate is the term for folic acid found in foods. Look for dark-green, leafy vegetables such as spinach, kale, dandelion greens, etc. Other good sources include asparagus, beets, beans, citrus fruits, broccoli, meat, and brewer's yeast.

DEFICIENCY

Deficiency of this vitamin is commonly found in alcoholics, pregnant women and people in nursing homes or those with absorption problems. Generally, folic acid deficiency produces few, if any, symptoms. It can however, cause depression, weakness, tiredness, and irritability. Because folic acid works with the neurotransmitter levels in your brain, depression is an understandable deficiency symptom.

DOSAGE

As with all water-soluble vitamins, what you don't use, you lose. However, very high doses, such as 15,000 mcg can cause problems with sleep, stomach problems and even seizures. You should stay around →**1,000 mcg** daily.

B12 - Cobalamins

The last of the B-vitamins we're going to study. It's water-soluble and naturally present in some foods.

As with the other B vitamins, B12 is required for red-blood-cell formation, DNA synthesis, and neurological function. It also works with energy production by converting carbohydrates, fats and protein into energy for the body to use. B12 is essential for the normal functioning of the brain, the nervous system and the formation of blood, and is involved in the metabolism of every cell in the body.

SOURCES

B12 is naturally found in animal products, and not usually present in plant foods. Meat, poultry, milk, fish, and milk products are major sources of this vitamin, while fortified breakfast cereals provide a good option for vegetarians.

DEFICIENCY

Most people consume enough vitamin B12, but you can become deficient. I would suggest that this vitamin be supplemented, particularly if you are over 50, or you take antacids on a regular basis.

Symptoms of deficiency include megaloblastic anemia, weakness, constipation, fatigue, loss of appetite, and weight loss. Numbness and tingling in the hands and feet can also occur. Additional symptoms include depression, confusion, dementia, poor memory, and difficulty maintaining balance.

In infants, signs of a B12 deficiency can include failure to thrive, movement disorders, developmental delays and anemia.

Most of the symptoms of B12 deficiency also apply to a B9 (folic acid) deficiency, so you should supplement both. A B12 deficiency can cause irreversible and severe damage, especially to the nervous system and the brain. It is VERY important to maintain adequate levels of this critical vitamin.

DOSAGE

B12 is not toxic, and can be tolerated in high doses by healthy individuals.

VITAMIN C

Vitamin C, or *ascorbic acid*, has probably had more publicity than any other vitamin. It has been called the miracle vitamin, offering cures for every disease. Ascorbic acid is an essential nutrient for the body, and an antioxidant, which protects the body from oxidative stress. We all should be taking it daily.

FREE RADICALS AND ANTIOXIDANTS

We have mentioned antioxidants before, but what exactly is an antioxidant? Antioxidants are reducing agents, and can limit the damage done by free radicals.

But what's a free radical? Atoms in our bodies have a center nucleus surrounded by pairs of smaller particles called electrons, similar to the planets in our solar system rotating around the sun. Sometimes one electron of a pair is lost, when the body converts food to energy, and the remaining one no longer behaves normally.

It is believed by many scientists that those unpaired electrons, called *free radicals*, cause enough damage that they're responsible for human aging. Free radicals cause damage to the cells and may be responsible for the development of cardiovascular disease and cancer, among other things. You are also exposed to free radical damage from the environment - cigarette smoke, air pollution and ultraviolet radiation from the sun.

Again, antioxidants can help reduce that damage. Whenever there are more free radicals in the body than antioxidants, it creates a condition known as *oxidative stress*. This has an impact on cardiovascular disease, hypertension, chronic inflammatory disease, diabetes, and IS also a factor in aging. Vitamin C is an antioxidant.

It's also a natural antihistamine, and works very well during colds to loosen nasal congestion. You would need at least 2,000 mg. daily for this effect.

LINUS PAULING

No work in Vitamin C would be complete without mentioning the works of Linus Pauling, two-time Nobel Prize winner. He researched Vitamin C extensively, and it was his theory that heart disease was caused by a chronic deficiency of vitamin C.

He wrote,

"Now I've got to the point where I think we can get almost complete control of cardiovascular disease, heart attacks and strokes. *The proper use of vitamin C and lysine can prevent cardiovascular disease and even cure it.*" [L. Pauling, 1994]

Much of his research has been ignored by the medical profession. But when you compare the money spent each year on 900,000 heart operations and angioplasties with Vitamin C and lysine, it doesn't take a brain surgeon to figure it out.

You can research his findings in more depth on the Internet, but here is a quote from one of his books.

"Hundreds of millions of dollars have been spent by the National Institutes of Health, the American Heart Association, and other agencies in support of studies of cardiovascular disease in relation to LDL and HDL cholesterol, triglycerides, saturated fats, and unsaturated fats. Very little attention has been paid to vitamin C and other vitamins. I think that these agencies have been betting on the wrong horse.

"It is fortunate that vitamin C is not a drug it is an orthomolecular substance, normally present in the human body and required for life, and it has extremely low toxicity. You do not need to have a physician's prescription or the approval of the medical establishment to use it in the best way to improve your health and to prevent heart disease. Your knowledge may even be greater and your judgment better than theirs." [Pauling, How to Live Longer and Feel Better, 1986]

Pauling also believed that *atherosclerosis*, or cardiovascular disease, is a natural healing process of the body, and that the walls of the veins and arteries are structurally weak from a deficiency of collagen, which is caused by inadequate vitamin C.

SOURCES

This vitamin is found in fresh fruits, berries and green vegetables. Most animals can make their own vitamin C, but Guinea pigs, apes and humans can't. This is another water-soluble vitamin, and we have to have a daily intake either from food or a supplement. Citrus fruits, such as oranges, lemons, limes, and grapefruit, are excellent sources.

Vitamin C works in almost all the functions of the body, but the tissues with the greatest percentage of vitamin C are the adrenal glands, pituitary, thymus, corpus luteum and retina. These have over 100 times the level in blood plasma.

DEFICIENCY

A deficiency will cause a disease called scurvy, a miserable problem in other centuries for sailors on ships out to sea. The gums bleed easily and wounds won't heal properly. After the discovery of vitamin C in 1928, it began to be used to stop scurvy in 1932.

DOSAGE

Linus Pauling recommends a dosage of →**3-6 grams (3,000 - 6,000 mg)** daily of Vitamin C and the same amount daily of L-Lysine. But tolerance to Vitamin C is an individual thing. The way to determine your tolerance is to take the vitamin C until you have diarrhea, and then back down on the dosage.

Maybe you'd better go take a dose of Vitamin C!

VITAMIN D

We may think of Vitamin D as being just one vitamin, but it is actually a fat-soluble group, consisting of D1, D2, D3, D4 and D5. Actually Vitamin D is not a vitamin, but a co-hormone. Whenever the skin is exposed to sunlight, Vitamin D (or *cholecalciferol*) is produced. It is then synthesized within the body, and not stored, as true vitamins are.

This vitamin helps our bodies produce normal levels of phosphorus and calcium, and is needed to properly absorb calcium, for maintaining strong bones. It can also inhibit high blood pressure and combat the growth of cancer cells. It strengthens our immune systems, and can really help us fight the common cold -- sometimes a dose at the onset can stop a cold in its tracks. Lack of Vitamin D in the winter months may well explain such high rates of the flu.

It may reduce the risk of developing multiple sclerosis. In the tropics, where there is much more sunlight, there is less frequency of multiple sclerosis, so this vitamin may be a factor.

Proper levels of Vitamin D may also help maintain the brain in later years. As we age, we are cautioned to stay out of the sun, but by doing so we deprive ourselves of this very important vitamin, which we need for proper brain function.

Vitamin D can reduce the severity of asthma, and reduce the risk of developing rheumatoid arthritis.

SOURCES

The very best source of Vitamin D is the sun. 10-20 minutes a day in sunlight (or even artificial light, such as a tanning bed) will produce a good level of Vitamin D3. Very few foods contain an abundant amount of this vitamin, and it's almost impossible to get enough through diet alone. Fatty fish, such as tuna or salmon are good sources, and supplements containing omega 3 oils (fish oil). Foods such as beef, cheese, eggs yolks, and liver contain small amounts, and food producers fortify our milk, cereal, and some breads with vitamin D.

DEFICIENCY

A deficiency of this vitamin can cause rickets in children and *osteoporosis* (porous bones) or *osteomalacia* (soft bones) in adults. Osteomalacia is a bone-thinning disorder characterized by muscle weakness and bone fragility. It contributes to chronic musculoskeletal pain. Older adults, people with dark skin or people using sunscreens are more prone to deficiency.

You can't overdose on the amount of Vitamin D **absorbed from the sun** because your body regulates its production; however, you *can* overdose on supplements. An overdose of Vitamin D will cause *hypercalcemia*, which produces symptoms of nausea, vomiting, weakness, nervousness, and ultimately renal failure. You can treat an overdose by discontinuing supplementation and restricting your calcium intake, although the kidney damage may be irreversible.

DOSAGE

How much do I need? The RDA is →**400 IU** daily for adults and children. If you are in the sunlight or a tanning bed you would want to lower the dose to about 200 IU or maybe even less, depending on your sun exposure. If you're not in the sun and are over the age of 50, you may want to increase the dosage to 600-800 IUs daily. Currently the "tolerable upper limit" is thought to be →**2,000 IU** per day. So you can play with your dose up to that limit, which should not produce any overdose symptoms.

Toxic overdose is a reality, but it's rare. Your risk of too little is far greater than your risk of overdose. Don't be afraid to supplement this very important vitamin. Foods contain low doses, and you won't overdose from food, nor will you overdose from the sun. The only way to overdose on Vitamin D is through supplementation.

VITAMIN E

Vitamin E is a family of *tocopherols* - alpha, beta, gamma and delta. It is a fat-soluble antioxidant, which protects cells from free radicals. Vitamin E can help minimize that damage.

Vitamin E supplements typically provide only alpha-tocopherol, but if you read the labels you might find a mixed supplement that contains the other tocopherols. There are a few out there. Synthetic alpha-tocopherol will be labeled as "dl" and is only half as active as the natural form, labeled "d." You would need twice as much of the supplement labeled "dl" as the natural form labeled "d."

Vitamin E is important in the formation of red blood cells and helps the body use Vitamin K. It also helps prevent cataracts, Alzheimer's disease, cancer, and heart disease.

It is important to take Vitamin E along with some form of oil or fat-containing food, either at a meal or with fish oil capsules. If you take Vitamin E on an empty stomach, your absorption is reduced by about 50%.

> →→ *Vitamin E can interfere with other medications - please see the CAUTIONS at the end of this section if you are taking other medications.*

SOURCES

Good sources include mustard greens, chard, sunflower seeds, turnip greens, almonds and spinach. Look for dark-green, leafy vegetables, nuts and oils.

DEFICIENCY

Vitamin E is found in a lot of foods, and it's fat-soluble, so your body will store it. A deficiency is rare, but if you are going to supplement, you should not take more than 400 IU daily.

DOSAGE

The maximum dosage of d-alpha for an adult would be →**1200 IU** daily. Because Vitamin E tends to thin the blood, a risk of bleeding with high doses can occur. The RDA is →**22.5 IU** daily for an adult.

If you have digestive problems, especially malabsorption, you can have an increased need for Vitamin E. Other events that may cause an increased need would be tingling or a loss of sensation in the arms, hands, legs, or feet, or if you experience liver or gallbladder problems.

VITAMIN E CAUTIONS

- Large doses of Vitamin E increase the risk of bleeding in individuals taking anticoagulant and antiplatelet medications, such as *Warfarin* (Coumadin). If you are taking this medication, **do not exceed →400 IU of Vitamin E daily.**

- If you are taking simvastatin (Zocor) or large doses of niacin, in combination with Vitamin E, Vitamin C, selenium, and beta-carotene (other antioxidants), it can cause a rise in the high-density lipoprotein (HDL), especially the HDL2, which is the most cardio-protective component.

- If you are undergoing cancer treatment, such as chemotherapy or radiotherapy you should avoid all antioxidant supplements. Antioxidant supplements, according to oncologists, inhibit damage in cancerous cells. This theory is still under investigation.

- Do not take supplements containing iron at the same time as Vitamin E.

VITAMIN K

Anyone who is on a blood-thinner has been told to stay away from this vitamin and any of the foods that contain it. I remember that a friend of mine was put on a blood-thinner by her doctor, who then told her she couldn't eat any green, leafy vegetables. But, by telling her that, he was causing her to miss out on a lot of really needed nutrients, and ultimately making her condition worse. Even with blood-thinner, you still need this very important vitamin. It's just like anything else - use common sense and moderation.

You need Vitamin K to maintain the cardiovascular system. It also promotes growth and development of bones, and will aid blood clotting. Vitamin K helps the heart get rid of excess calcium, which protects you from atherosclerosis, calcium deposits that clog important arteries and block the circulation of blood. It might just save you from that bypass surgery!

SOURCES

Vitamin K is contained in green, leafy vegetables, eggs and soybeans. Parsley is a good way to get your daily dose of Vitamin K - two tablespoons contain 153% of the RDA.

DEFICIENCY

A deficiency of Vitamin K can cause cystic fibrosis, irritable bowel syndrome, and many digestive problems. If you have digestive problems, you need to include this very important vitamin in your diet. Research has shown that people suffering from Alzheimer's disease have a deficiency of Vitamin K. It also protects the liver and spleen from cancer, and helps diabetics and obese people by regulating insulin in the body. By working with calcium, supplementation of this vitamin may delay the development of osteoporosis.

The common signs of Vitamin K deficiency are heavy menstrual bleeding, gum bleeding, nose bleeding and easy bruising. Bleeding can also occur in the digestive tract, and blood may appear in the urine. Other symptoms include prolonged clotting times, hemorrhaging and anemia.

It is very important to supplement this vitamin during pregnancy, as it helps in the overall development of the fetus.

DOSAGE

Dosage is →**65-80 mg** daily. There is no known toxicity with high doses, although people on blood thinners do need to watch their intake.

HEALTHY CHOICES

IN AN *UNHEALTHY* WORLD

CHAPTER 6

MINERALS

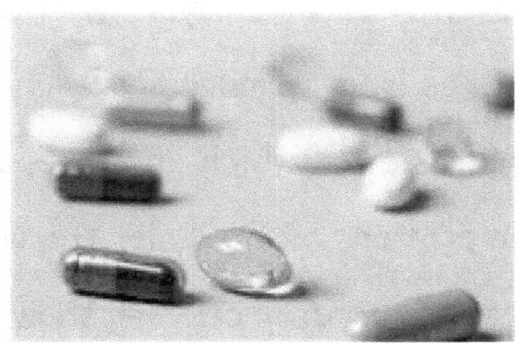

MINERALS

Vitamins are critical, but without minerals, you simply can't utilize them! And you have to *consume* them in food or supplements, because your body can manufacture a few vitamins, but not a single mineral. So a mineral deficiency is much more likely to occur than a vitamin deficiency.

Minerals are essential to life. They are crucial for many of the body's functions, such as keeping the blood and the fluid in the tissues from becoming too acidic or alkaline, transporting oxygen, normalizing the nervous system, and maintaining and repairing tissues and bone.

Checking your mineral levels periodically is extremely important, and can be done simply with a hair analysis. (See Chapter 7) Imagine a hair like tree rings - it has long-term memory. Any toxins, heavy metals or drug and chemical residues which are present in the body are embedded in the fiber proteins of the hair. The way all of your glands, such as adrenals and thyroid, are functioning shows up in the hair.

It's the ideal medium for testing -- a two-inch strand can provide a four-month history of the elements inside the body, giving us a comprehensive picture of what's going on.

In the following chapters we'll take a look at the broad range of essential minerals and toxic elements that a hair analysis reports.

CALCIUM

I'm sure most of us have heard a lot about calcium. Doctors are always telling their patients to *take calcium*, commercials are telling you to *take calcium* for strong bones and teeth, *calcium*, *calcium* -- you hear it everywhere!

But what exactly *is* calcium, and what does it do in the body? First of all, it's essential to every living creature. As a matter of fact, calcium is the most abundant *metal* in many animals.

About 1% of the body's calcium is used for muscle function, nerve transmission, and the operation of veins and arteries. The other 99% is for the bones and teeth. Bone is constantly re-forming and making new bone, and the calcium is used here. As you age, old bone can break down faster than new bone forms, and you can develop osteoporosis.

But calcium can be tricky! In some of my clients who actually have osteoporosis or bone loss, I still see elevated calcium levels. How can this be?

When the thyroid and adrenals are not operating at full-tilt, the calcium doesn't go where it is supposed to -- bones and teeth. Instead, it's deposited in the soft tissues, where it "overdoses" and causes trouble -- the gallbladder (gallstones), kidneys (kidney stones), arteries (hardening of the arteries). You have to give the thyroid and adrenals a boost to get that calcium where it belongs.

SOURCES

Milk, cheese, yogurt, and the dairy products. Other sources are kale, broccoli, and dark green leafy vegetables. Some foods are fortified with calcium, such as fruit juices and cereals. "Tums" and "Rolaids" also contain calcium. But you *should* get your calcium from food, because the body recognizes it easily.

DOSAGE

Generally, it's the same for men and women, except for pregnant or lactating women (they could safely double it).

- Anyone over the age of 4 normally needs →1,000 - 1,300 mg daily.
- During the teenage years you should raise the dose to →1,300 mg. This is the time when our children usually have their "growth spurts," and the need for calcium is greater.

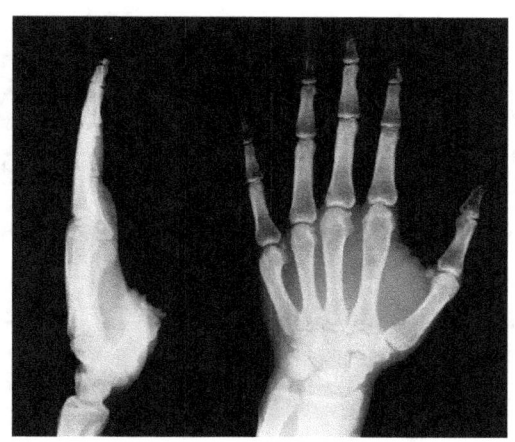

MAGNESIUM

Some minerals must maintain a balance with others for optimal health, and calcium's best friend is magnesium. Actually, it is more like a "love-hate" relationship. This partnership isn't fully understood, but we know magnesium is required for calcium to play an ideal role in your metabolism. At the same time, magnesium can compete with calcium and prevent its triggering certain activities, such as contraction of a muscle, or a relay of a nerve message. Magnesium also has a strong relationship with potassium.

Two thirds of all of our magnesium is in our bones, or actually, on the *surface* of the bones. If the body needs additional magnesium, it can simply pull it from there. Magnesium doesn't help in *building* bone -- it just rests on the surface like a lattice, giving them structure.

Magnesium is the "smooth" mineral that causes our muscles to relax. This can be beneficial for the heart, as well as any muscle spasms you might have. It's also used in the treatment of headaches, and can be a lifesaver for migraine sufferers. The role of magnesium is very diverse, and a deficiency will affect every body system.

DOSAGE

The upper limit was set by the National Academy of Science at →350 milligrams a day. If you take too much, you'll have diarrhea. Magnesium toxicity can also cause generalized symptoms, such as increased drowsiness or weakness.

Generally, it's hard to overdose on magnesium, especially from food sources. Excess magnesium is eliminated through the kidneys, so if you have a kidney problem, magnesium could accumulate to high levels. Or, if you consume a lot of Epsom Salts or Milk of Magnesia, you could have high levels.

SOURCES

Magnesium is present in so many foods it would be hard to list them all here. Some good ones are spinach, Swiss chard, squash, broccoli, mustard greens, pumpkin seeds, peppermint, and turnip greens.

PHOSPHORUS

Phosphorus is required by every cell in the body. It makes up 1% of a person's total weight, but is found mainly in the bones and teeth, since its main function is their formation. It also helps in utilizing fats and carbohydrates, and in the maintenance and repair of cells and tissues. It's essential for the storage of ATP, which is a molecule the body uses to store energy.

Phosphorus works with the B-vitamins, contraction of muscles, function of the kidneys, nerve conduction and the regularity of the heartbeat.

DOSAGE

About →**700 mg** a day for adults is a good dose.

SOURCES

Phosphorus is found in almost all foods, because it is so essential for health. This is a mineral you usually don't have to supplement because it is so readily available.

SODIUM/POTASSIUM

These are two minerals which must stay in balance. Too much or too little of either can cause you problems.

SODIUM

Sodium is used in the body to regulate blood pressure and also blood volume. It is also critical for the functioning of the muscles and the nerves. Too much sodium can cause elevated blood pressure and fluid retention.

POTASSIUM

The proper functioning of the heart, kidneys, muscles, nerves and digestive system all depend on potassium. Potassium works with the regulation of the heartbeat and the function of the muscles. Too much or too little will profoundly affect the nervous system and may cause irregular, and sometimes dangerous, heartbeats.

Sodium and potassium both help with communication between the brain, nerves, nervous systems and the muscles. Both sodium and potassium are also involved with the adrenal and thyroid glands. Sodium has more to do with the adrenal, and potassium with the thyroid gland.

SOURCES

You usually get all the potassium you need from the foods you eat.

We all know that our main source of sodium is salt. But sodium also occurs naturally in most foods, including drinking water. Processed foods and fast food usually contain high amounts of sodium.

Although we look first at the salt shaker when trying to lower our sodium levels, actual salt intake is secondary. The main causes of imbalance trace back to stress or anger, a zinc or magnesium deficiency, or toxic metals in the system.

But I would still recommend that you not consume table salt. Sea salt and Himalayan crystal salt are much healthier.

COPPER / ZINC

Here are two more minerals that must stay in balance, and once again, too much or too little can be really hard on your health.

Zinc determines how much copper is stored in the body. If you have a deficiency of zinc, too much copper builds up in the tissues. The balance of these two minerals will determine the rate of the thyroid hormone production. Copper slows the thyroid, and zinc increases its activity. Hyperthyroidism (too fast) and hypothyroidism (too slow) appear to be stages in the same disease. Probably both are caused by nutrient deficiencies. Whenever hyperthyroidism exists the deficiencies become more severe.

COPPER

Copper aids in your absorption of iron, works with the thyroid, and supplies oxygen to the blood. It's a brain stimulant, a natural yeast-fighter, parallels estrogen levels and helps to oxidize vitamin C. These are just a *few* of its functions in the body.

The standard dosage should be about →**700 mcg** a day for a 7-13 year old, →**890 mcg** a day for 14-18 year old and adults about →**900 mcg** a day. Usually you get enough copper from your diet.

SOURCES

Copper is found in an abundance of foods, including fruits, whole grains, leafy green vegetables, organ meats, poultry, nuts, and dark chocolate.

DOSAGE

This isn't something to take haphazardly. Copper toxicity can cause migraine headaches, cancer, arthritis symptoms, depression, liver degeneration, and hair loss, just to name a few. Excessive copper in children can signal ADHD, ADD and ear infections.

ZINC

Zinc works with your immune system, normal tissue growth and repair, and cell reproduction. If you feel a cold coming on, start supplementing zinc. It will shorten the duration of the cold, and zinc lozenges are wonderful for sore throat pain.

Zinc also helps increase progesterone and lower estrogen levels.

SOURCES

Meat, liver, eggs, milk, whole grains, seafood and many other foods contain zinc.

DOSAGE

Children over 14 and adults need →**11mg** daily. A good way to check your zinc levels is to look at your fingernails: if you have white spots on them, you're low in zinc. If there are no white spots, you probably don't need to supplement zinc.

Zinc toxicity will interfere with your copper metabolism and will reduce your iron function. You may have abdominal pain, vomiting, headache, dizziness and irritability.

IRON

Iron is essential to most life forms. It aids in the formation of red blood cells, which transport oxygen to the tissues.

There are two kinds of dietary iron: "heme" and "nonheme." Heme iron is found in animal foods, such as red meats, fish and poultry, which originally contained hemoglobin.

Iron found in plant foods, such as beans and greens, is referred to as nonheme iron. Whenever you find an iron-enriched food, this is the type of iron that has been added. Heme iron is absorbed better, but most dietary iron is the non-heme variety.

Iron deficiency is considered to be the number one nutritional disorder in the world by the World Health Organization. They say that as many as 80% of the world's population may be deficient in iron.

Adult men and postmenopausal women are often exceptions, though, and will generally have enough iron from food sources. They should not take supplements containing iron, since it can accumulate in the body and become toxic.

A good dosage for iron is about →**8 mg** a day until you reach the age of 50 -- after that you don't need to supplement iron.

MANGANESE

Manganese is present in small amounts in the body. It is mainly found in the bones, kidneys, liver and pancreas. This mineral helps the body to form connective tissue and strong bones, helps the blood to clot and aids in the production of sex hormones. It also works with metabolizing fat and carbohydrates, blood sugar regulation and the absorption of calcium. And it's necessary for nerve function and normal brain activity.

SOURCES

Manganese is found in whole grains, nuts and seeds, and most Americans don't get enough in their diet, because the typical American diet contains more refined grains instead of whole grains. Refined grains contain much less manganese.

DOSAGE

Manganese is necessary for strong bones. If you have osteoporosis, you would want to take a combination of manganese, calcium, zinc, and copper, as these are the main minerals that build strong bones. It can also be helpful with arthritis pain.

The symptoms of premenstrual syndrome have been helped by supplementing manganese in their diet. Studies have found that supplementing manganese has helped with mood swings and cramps.

Manganese has also been used in the treatment of epilepsy. People with seizures have shown lower manganese levels in their blood.

A deficiency, or even just low levels, can cause infertility, malformation of bones and seizures. People with diabetes usually have low levels of manganese in their blood. Manganese works with the pancreas and this is where the insulin is produced. Maybe there is a connection.

But too much manganese can cause an abnormal concentration in the brain, and lead to neurological disorders resembling Parkinson's disease.

→**3.5 to 7 mg** a day is a suggested dose.

CHROMIUM

Chromium is a mineral we need in small amounts. Exactly what it does and how much it takes aren't well defined, but it is known to enhance the action of insulin, and is directly involved in carbohydrate, fat and protein metabolism.

SOURCES

Many foods, such as meat, whole grains, fruits and vegetables, contain very small amounts. Foods that are high in simple sugars are generally low in chromium.

DOSAGE

You can become deficient in chromium by eating a lot of processed foods, insufficient B5, iron overload, or gastrointestinal dysfunction. Effects of deficiency include hyperglycemia, fatigue, elevated LDL cholesterol, diabetes-like symptoms, and a risk of cardiovascular disease.

A good suggested dose is →100-400 mcg a day. High levels of chromium are not very toxic, but they can cause bad dreams or insomnia.

SELENIUM

Selenium is another mineral required in small amounts, about →**55 mcgs** a day. It is an antioxidant, which will help prevent cellular damage from free radicals. (Page 87) It also helps regulate thyroid function and plays an important role in the immune system. And selenium can bind and inactivate mercury.

SOURCES

Plant foods, meat and sea foods are dietary choices for this mineral. A deficiency is rare, and most cases are associated with severe gastrointestinal problems, such as Crohn's disease.

BORON

Boron is vital for bone health, and needed for bone density. If you are postmenopausal, boron supplementation is critical in keeping calcium and magnesium in the bone. It is also needed to balance levels of estrogen.

SOURCES

You can get boron from soaps, cleaners, and certain medications. Food sources are apples, bananas, celery, almonds, beans, broccoli, avocados and most other fruits and vegetables.

DOSAGE

High levels are non-toxic, but that doesn't mean you should have high levels.

A balanced diet should provide all the boron that you will need but if you would like to supplement for bone health you could safely add →**6 mg** daily to your diet.

COBALT

Cobalt is a trace mineral that is stored mainly in the liver. It helps form vitamin B-12, and may play a role in treating anemia that doesn't respond well to any other treatment. It contributes to formation of red blood cells, and may also help with fatigue and digestive disorders.

SOURCES

Cobalt is found in dairy products, liver, meats, and most foods containing vitamin B-12.

DOSAGE

You only need small amounts of this mineral, and a deficiency is extremely rare. If you do become deficient, you won't be able to manufacture B-12, and that could lead to pernicious anemia.

You'll probably get enough cobalt from a healthy diet, but it is safe to supplement at →**1.4 mg** a day.

MOLYBDENUM

This mineral is needed for normal growth and development. It may protect teeth and enhance iron absorption. Molybdenum becomes a part of the bones, liver and kidneys.

SOURCES

Sources include beans, whole grains, cereals, peas, lean meats.

DOSAGE

Deficiency symptoms are rare, as you usually get adequate amounts from your diet. Generally, the only people that need to supplement this mineral are people who have had severe burns or are extremely ill and being fed intravenously or with a NG tube.

Excess molybdenum will cause a drop in copper, but you could supplement at →**43 mcg**. daily.

SULFUR

Sulfur is one mineral that has no proven deficiency symptoms. It aids bile secretion in the liver, and aids in your metabolism. It may also improve arthritis symptoms and help protect you against toxic substances.

SOURCES

Most people will get the necessary amount of sulfur from a good diet. Natural sources include beans, eggs, fish, milk, garlic and lean beef and meats.

DOSAGE

Large quantities of sulfur are required for health, but there is no RDA. Sulfur is obtained from, and it is used for, amino acids. You should have an adequate intake if you eat enough protein.

ADDITIONAL MINERALS

The following minerals are also tested in a hair analysis, but their levels are not as important as those listed above. For the best health, you should have them, as well as the above minerals, all in normal levels.

GERMANIUM

This mineral boosts oxygenation of the cells. It also helps the immune system and helps to rid the body of toxins and poisons. It has been used to treat rheumatoid arthritis, food allergies, and candidiasis.

Sources include garlic and onions.

No proven deficiency symptoms exist.

BARIUM

If you have ever had to drink that horrible white stuff that tastes like liquid chalk, in preparation for an x-ray, you know what Barium is.

Barium can be toxic in large doses so it good to have your levels checked periodically.

BISMUTH

Whenever you have feelings of depression and tiredness, and you don't know why, it can be caused by an element imbalance. It could be bismuth.

It has a low toxicity, but since it has many uses, it is a very common element in many homes. Bismuth is found in products used to treat diarrhea and upset stomachs. It is also found in many cosmetics, particularly lipstick.

With a mild toxicity you might experience constipation or irritable bowels, bad breath, or just not feeling well. High levels can cause memory loss, tremors, dementia, and protein loss through the urine.

RUBIDIUM

Rubidium is a benign mineral that typically parallels the potassium level, and is more important for plants than humans. It can form an oxide which will irritate the adrenal glands, raising the sodium levels. This can help rebalance a very ill person.

It is found in many common foods - meats and vegetables.

LITHIUM

Lithium is one of the essential body elements, a very important nutrient for development of the brain and hormones.

The natural lithium found in foods is very different from the pharmaceutical lithium used to treat bi-polar disorder. If your natural lithium levels are low you may experience mood swings, PMS, or depression.

Lithium is found in greens, kelp, seafood and sea vegetables.

High levels can cause dermatitis, hypotension, low sodium levels, confusion, edema and nausea. Lithium will also compete with calcium and magnesium.

NICKEL

Nickel is required in very low amounts. It can hyper-sensitize the immune system, and cause an allergic reaction to many substances.

High levels of nickel can be toxic to the kidneys and may even cause cancer. Nickel is one of the elements contained in cigarette smoke. Symptoms of long term exposure include dermatitis, chronic rhinitis, and liver problems.

PLATINUM

This mineral is usually absorbed through inhalation. It is very rare, and most exposures are from occupational sources. It can cause COPD, wheezing, water retention, and elevated cholesterol.

THALLIUM

This mineral is highly toxic, and should be in the same category as lead and mercury. Sources of thallium include tobacco, cement dust, and some fertilizers.

Symptoms may appear long after the exposure, and include sleep disturbances, kidney dysfunction, cardiac and liver stress.

VANADIUM

Vanadium has direct effects on thyroid metabolism and also on insulin production. It is a blood sugar nutrient, and also assists in the regulating potassium and sodium.

Sources include liver, radishes, nuts and fish. Excess levels can be toxic, and some symptoms are bronchitis, kidney failure, diarrhea and decreased appetite.

STRONTIUM

Strontium is one of the essential bone nutrients, similar to calcium and boron. It can even replace calcium in some biological processes.

It's found in cereals, grains, dairy products and seafood.

If your levels of strontium and calcium are high in the hair, then they are typically low in the bones, showing that the bones aren't assimilating nutrients properly. This can be associated with a lack of vitamin C.

TIN

This is a very toxic element, and levels of tin usually accumulate from environmental exposure. Sources include dental fillings, cosmetics, and some food and beverage containers.

Some of the symptoms of high levels are muscle weakness, skin irritation, anemia, GI tract irritation.

Tin will usually make a ball in the body, and form a cyst.

TITANIUM

This is the metal so popular in the energy bracelets. Great for energy, but not so much inside the body. The dust from titanium, when inhaled, has been classified as carcinogenic to humans.

A lot of sunscreens contain small particles of titanium, which are absorbed into the skin. The effects of titanium on human health are not very well understood yet.

TUNGSTEN

You can be exposed to tungsten either through natural processes or human industrial activities, by breathing air that contains the dust or by eating food or drinking water contaminated with it.

High levels of tungsten can produce skin, eye, throat, or nose irritation. Chronic exposure can cause lung problems such as shortness of breath, coughing and wheezing.

ZIRCONIUM

Zirconium has a low toxicity level, and usually passes through the gut without being absorbed. If any *is* absorbed, it tends to accumulate more in the skeleton than in tissue. So if your levels are high on the hair analysis, there might be an even higher concentration in the bones.

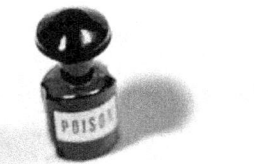

TOXIC ELEMENTS

In a hair analysis we also check for toxic elements. These are present in our environment in the air, soil, water, plants, and animals, and these metals end up posing a health threat. The body has a protective device, whenever you are exposed to a toxin: it pulls the toxin out of the blood and deposits it in the tissues. This is why so many of our metal exposures don't show up in a blood test, but they can be found in a tissue sample, like the hair.

Metals can cause all kinds of consequences, depending on the amount, the length of time and the health of the individual. A lot of them could have been with you all of your life. They don't just leave of their own accord -- you have to take steps to remove them from the body.

In our pollutant-filled environment, exposure occurs through day-to-day living. It comes from cigarette smoke, antiperspirants, antacids, cans, tap water, tooth fillings, and fish, not to mention things you would never expect, like jewelry, make-up and even dietary supplements.

ANTIMONY

Hair is the ideal medium for testing antimony exposure. You may still have elevated levels as long as a year after exposure.

Some consider it more toxic than arsenic, while others disagree. It is usually excreted in the urine and feces.

Antimony affects liver functions, possibly interferes with sulfur chemistry, and can impair enzymes. Symptoms may vary, and can include fatigue, muscle aches and inflammation, hypotension, immune system dysfunction, and angina. Later symptoms can include kidney failure. If it is absorbed through the skin, you can have "antimony spots," looking very much like chicken pox.

The usual sources of antimony are food and smoking, though some gunpowder also may contain antimony. It is also used in the manufacture of paints, glass, solder, and batteries.

URANIUM

Most exposure comes from the natural uranium in ground and drinking water. It is also present in root vegetables and high-phosphate fertilizers. Uranium mostly accumulates in the kidneys and bones, but also in the liver and the spleen.

The main symptom of uranium is chronic fatigue. More severe exposure can result in kidney failure and all forms of cancer.

ARSENIC

Arsenic is thought to be essential, in trace amounts, but is extremely poisonous. It is a carcinogen, and raises the risk of skin, liver lymphatic and lung cancer.

Some sources of arsenic are tap water, rat poisons, seafood, air pollution, and wine.

It deposits in the hair, skin, nails, thyroid gland, bones and in the gastrointestinal tract. Symptoms of exposure include headaches, confusion, changes in fingernail color, diarrhea, convulsions, vomiting, blood in urine, hair loss, confusion, and drowsiness. Chronic exposure will cause problems for the nervous system, the cardiovascular system, and the lymphatic system.

Arsenic is easier to remove from the body than some of the other metals because it is lighter in composition.

BERYLLIUM

Beryllium is toxic to both humans and animals. It is antagonistic to magnesium, and can cause immune dysfunction, rickets and damage the liver, kidneys, lungs and skin.

It's poorly absorbed through the intestines, but easily absorbed by the skin and lungs. Usually inhalation is the route of exposure.

Sources are tobacco, optical lens coatings, electronic components.

MERCURY

Mercury poisoning has probably made the news more than any other heavy metal. We are concerned about our dental fillings and the vaccines we give our children.

In the past we were careless with mercury. I remember the old mercury thermometers -- if you dropped one and it broke, you just picked up the glass and the little balls of mercury and went on. What we didn't know was that the little balls of mercury were very harmful to our health. When I was a little girl, my best friend's mother dropped a thermometer and picked up the mercury with her hands. Her gold rings temporarily turned a silver color -- just imagine what it did to her body.

Mercury can mimic multiple sclerosis (MS). Before you accept treatment for this disease from your doctor, please check your mercury levels. Mercury works in the nervous system and causes tremors and mood swings. High levels can also cause kidney damage, hormonal imbalances, numbness in the extremities, loss of coordination, confusion, phobias, fatigue, anxiety, and depression. Mercury poisoning can go undetected for years because the symptoms aren't particularly noticeable -- you just think it's stress or other minor illnesses.

Common sources of mercury include dental fillings, adhesives, cosmetics, diuretics, vaccines, seafood, tattoos, paints, broken thermometers, and mercurochrome.

CADMIUM

Cadmium is a very toxic metal, and has no metabolic function in the body. It will accumulate in the body and replace your stores of zinc in the liver and kidneys. It will also affect the lungs, arteries, heart, testes, and bones.

Cigarette smoke contains cadmium, and smokers usually have high amounts in their tissues. High levels can cause high blood pressure, hair loss, joint stiffness and soreness, anemia, and an altered sense of smell.

Common sources include batteries, ceramics, coffee, tea, hair treatments, motor oil, silver polish, colas, fumes from burning tires, rubber and plastics, welding materials and fertilizers.

LEAD

Lead can be very serious for both children and adults. It is retained in the nervous system, bones, glands, and brain. Lead will also interfere with the metabolism of Vitamin D. Children with learning disabilities or ADHD/ADD usually have high levels of lead. If your child exhibits any symptoms of learning disabilities, it is very important to get them tested.

A blood test won't show long-term lead exposure, but only ongoing or recent exposure. Your body, once again, uses its protective devices and pulls the lead out of the blood and deposits it in the tissues.

Sources of lead include auto exhaust, car batteries, canned fruit and juice, leaded gasoline, lead crystal dishes, lead water pipes, paint, and mascara.

Lead can affect the body's ability to use calcium, magnesium and zinc. High levels can cause anemia, headaches, fatigue, weight loss, memory loss, constipation, and insomnia.

ALUMINUM

Aluminum is found in so many things we use on a common basis, such as cans, cookware, aluminum foil, antacids, baking powder, cigarette filters, deodorants, drinking water, milk products, tobacco smoke, pesticides, table salt, and toothpaste.

Almost everyone has a piece of aluminum cookware in their kitchen. Unfortunately, aluminum can leach out of the cookware and be deposited in the brain and nervous system. It has been linked to Alzheimer's disease and dementia.

Children and adults with low zinc and learning disorders such as ADD, ADHD and autism usually have high levels of aluminum. It can also cause high levels of ammonia in your tissues, which can lead to kidney problems or even dialysis.

Symptoms include fatigue, headache, forgetfulness, loss of balance, and colic. It can also lead to osteoporosis and symptoms similar to Alzheimer's.

HEALTHY CHOICES
IN AN *UNHEALTHY* WORLD

CHAPTER 7
NATURAL HEALING CHOICES

How a Naturopathic Doctor Can Help

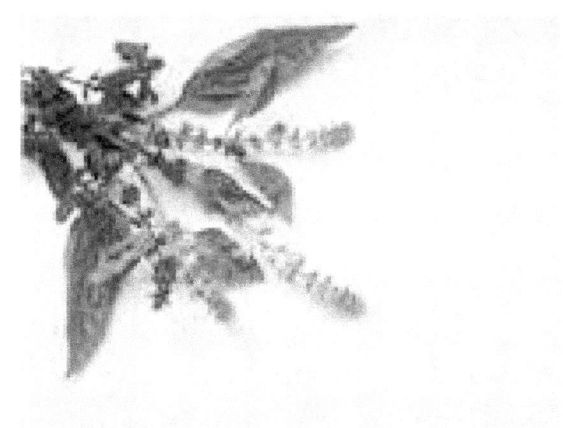

What is Naturopathy?
What does a Naturopathic Physician do?

The word "naturopathy" comes from Greek roots, and means "treating a disease by natural means." And that's what a Naturopathic Physician tries to do, guided by 6 basic principles:

1. Nature's healing power

We believe that the body has an innate healing ability. Clients are taught to use diet, exercise, lifestyle changes and natural therapies to ward off and combat disease. We look at the whole person and take a complete history. A person is not a tumor or a heart attack, and doesn't want to be treated that way.

2. Identify the cause of disease and treat it, not just the symptoms.

Unless you find the true cause of the illness, you are just covering-up symptoms. My job is to try to find the root of the problem, and stop it at its source.

3. Do no harm.

The safety of my clients is my utmost concern. Healing compounds used in my practice, such as dietary supplements, herbal extracts, and homeopathy have little or no side effects. A Naturopath does no invasive procedures, such as shots or surgery. Each diagnosis and treatment is personally designed for that client. Each person is unique, and heals differently.

4. Treat the whole person, not just the symptoms.

Once again each individual is different and needs to be treated differently. A medical problem does not just happen -- it develops over time in response to conditions in a person's life, and the treatment needs to address that issue. Get to the root of the problem and fix it!

5. The physician becomes a teacher.

A Naturopath teaches clients how to eat, relax, and exercise in the healthiest ways, and will also teach them to nurture themselves both physically and emotionally. We teach self-responsibility, and stay in close contact with the clients.

6. Prevention of illness

"An ounce of prevention is worth a pound of cure" is a very true statement. Preventive medicine will save money, pain and even lives.

WHAT TYPES OF ILLNESS DO NATUROPATHS TREAT?

A Naturopath can help with any illness. We use non-invasive procedures for diagnosis and treatment. Natural medicine can work with anything from the most minor ailment to the most serious. Any illness can be helped with improvement in diet and some lifestyle changes.

NATUROPATHIC HEALING TECHNIQUES

There are many aspects of natural health, but I have found that some work better for me than others. Those are the ones I prefer to use in my practice, and the ones we'll explore in this book. I have tested and tried them all.

HAIR ANALYSIS

A hair-tissue mineral analysis is an analytical test which measures the mineral content of the hair. Studies show that hair may be a more appropriate tissue than blood or urine for studying exposure to some elements, because the body has a protective device that, when exposed to toxins, will pull them out of the blood and deposit them in the tissues, making hair the perfect medium.

Hair can show mineral status and toxic metal accumulation from long term or even acute exposure. The Environmental Protection Agency uses hair testing in determining toxic metal exposure. Besides industrial contamination, heavy metals are picked up through cigarette smoke, dental fillings, aluminum cookware, and many other things that we are exposed to on a daily basis. You could have even picked up heavy metals from the time spent in the womb. If you never took steps to remove them, they're still with you. They don't leave the body of their own accord – you have to help.

Not only do you test for toxic metals, but also for minerals. Minerals can sometimes be more important than vitamins in metabolic functions. The body can produce vitamins, but it cannot produce minerals or get rid of the excesses.

Some examples:

- Zinc is necessary for growth hormones, and works with the production, storage and secretion of insulin;

- Potassium is essential for transporting nutrients into the cells;

- Sodium is associated with hypertension, but you still need sodium for normal health.

These minerals must be in proper balance to function as they should. Many factors can cause an imbalance, such as diet, stress, medications, pollution, improper use of nutritional supplements, or inherited patterns. Mineral imbalances will not correct themselves.

Hair is an ideal tissue for testing. It can be cut easily and sent to the lab without special handling requirements. You collect a small sample of hair (about 1 teaspoon) from the first inch-and-a-half of growth on the scalp. It should be taken from various places all over your head. It is then sent to the lab to undergo testing. The only requirement is that you don't use medicated shampoos, such as Head and Shoulders, which can affect the results of the test.

Your hair grows approximately 1 inch per month, so a sample can show what's going on with your body within the last month.

Although hair analysis doesn't check vitamin levels directly, it's still a good indicator of your vitamin status. Minerals and vitamins work together. For instance, vitamin C affects iron absorption and will reduce copper retention. Therefore, if you detect copper and/or low iron, you need to look at your vitamin C. Vitamin B1 enhances sodium retention and Vitamin A enhances the utilization of zinc.

A hair analysis will also show how your thyroid and adrenal glands are functioning. Indirectly, it will show your hormone levels. For example, zinc helps to increase progesterone levels and lower estrogen. Copper corresponds with elevated estrogen. If one of these is out of balance, so are your hormones. These are just a few reasons why a hair analysis is so important.

The lab that I use for hair analysis gives a very comprehensive report. It may include glandular extracts, vitamin/mineral recommendations and a special diet, depending on your results. Each report contains about 10 pages, detailing your analysis. I have had people tell me they've never seen anything hit the nail on the head like this before.

I would highly recommend that you have one, especially if you've had problems the doctor couldn't pinpoint.

HERBOLOGY

What would a natural health practitioner be without the use of herbs? Herbs are one of our first weapons in the fight against disease. According to the "Doctrine of Signatures," plants contain a "signature" which can tell you how to use the plant. For instance, dandelions, which everyone tries to kill, are yellow. Bile is yellow; therefore, these are good for cleaning the gallbladder and liver.

Herbal remedies can often be taken in many different ways -- the fresh herb, dried herb, tincture, or tea. You may just simply add some fresh herb to a salad, or you may want a particular dosage that requires a tincture or capsule form.

Anytime you can get fresh herbs it's better to do so, but they're sometimes hard to get when you need them. You may, for instance, need parsley root in the winter. Parsley root removes excess water from the body, and people with edema may need to use it year-round. Then you have to rely on capsules or tinctures.

Dried herbs can be used many different ways. You may use them to formulate your tinctures, in cooking, or in a tea. Drinking an herbal tea is the weakest form of use.

Herbs are very versatile and can be used in many different ways. But people have a tendency to assume that, because herbs are natural, they can use them indiscriminately. I've heard the statement, "It's natural, so it can't hurt you."

But you have to remember that herbs are *medicines*, and you have herbs safe enough even for a newborn baby, and then you have much stronger herbs -- to be used with caution, and only when absolutely necessary. It's very important to know the difference!

You should not try to medicate yourself. I knew of a case that could have turned out badly. There was an older lady with a heart problem who took ginger, which is very good for the heart. Ginger is a fairly safe herb, but the lady's blood pressure went through the roof. Of course she stopped taking it, and suffered no damage, but an herbalist with advanced training would know that ginger is also a stimulant, and will raise the blood pressure. It could have caused a heart attack or stroke.

Herbs are extremely valuable medicine - just make sure you get the advice of a certified herbalist.

HOMEOPATHY

Homeopathy is a widely-used form of alternative medicine, based on the idea that the body will heal itself, given the opportunity. It was developed in Germany more than 200 years ago, and has been practiced in the United States since the 19th century. Homeopathy is absolutely safe for all ages. All remedies are derived from natural substances.

"Like cures like" is the homeopathic principle. This means that certain substances that will produce symptoms of a disease in *healthy people* will cure someone that *has that disease.* It sounds funny to many of us, but it works like this:

A small amount of a substance is taken and diluted, then shaken vigorously. This is called "potentization." It is believed to transmit energy from the original substance to the final remedy.

Then that mixture is further diluted, and shaken again. It may be diluted repeatedly. Each time it is diluted it is shaken vigorously.

Most homeopathic remedies have been diluted so many times that chemical testing can find none of the original substance remaining. However, these are some of the most potent remedies, because homeopathy works in reverse to what we're used to with conventional medicine: the more dilute the remedy, the stronger the effect.

Remedies are in various strengths; for instance, a 30C is medium-strength. You'll probably see them marked "6X" or "30C." Typically you won't find the higher strengths; these would need to be prescribed.

The "X" represents 10, and means that the potency is based on the ratio of 1 part substance to 10 parts dilution. These are considered low potencies, and are often used for children or first-aid treatment. They can be given as often as every 10 minutes until the symptoms subside.

The "C" represents 100, and means that the potency is based on the ratio of 1 part substance to 99 parts dilution. These are medium potencies, and are used for the more chronic problems. They are usually given every hour until the symptoms subside.

Whenever you take a homeopathic remedy, most of the time it works immediately. If you are taking it for an injury, it may take longer.

There are homeopathic remedies for every ailment you can think of, and these can be very specific.

It's almost impossible to find a true homeopathic physician in the United States anymore. A true homeopath would sit down with you and take your life history for a couple of hours. After analyzing this information, he would narrow the remedy choices down to one that best fit you.

Most homeopaths now use combinations. If you choose the wrong remedy, it simply will have no effect on you. Absolutely nothing will happen. So the combinations are safe for anyone. For instance, if you had a cold, you would choose a combination remedy for the cold. It would consist of about 10-15 remedies targeted for colds. One or more of them would work for you, and the others would have no effect.

When you take a remedy, you don't eat or drink anything for 15 minutes prior or 15 minutes afterward. The remedies are very easy to take: Simply place the remedy under your tongue for about 30 seconds, if a liquid form, or hold the tablets under your tongue until they dissolve. When you've chosen the right remedy, you'll feel relaxed and may even fall asleep.

Homeopathic remedies work wonders for young children. They work on colic, ear infections, stomachaches, etc. My grandson used to refer to them as happy pills because they'd make him feel so much better. You don't have to worry about any side effects or dangerous reactions.

We always keep Arnica 200C in our medicine chest for injuries. It will minimize pain and bruising, and you'll heal very quickly.

As I mentioned earlier, homeopathic remedies are extremely safe. The only side effect is that liquid remedies are processed in alcohol, which allows them to get into your bloodstream more quickly. So you need caution in giving these to small children.

Once again, please don't try to medicate yourself. Homeopathic remedies are used for many different ailments, and you should seek someone who is qualified in dispensing these remedies.

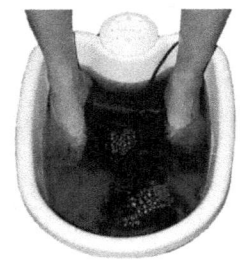

ION FOOT DETOX

Many years ago it was discovered that whenever the body is more acidic, you are sick more often. An ion cleanse will change the polarity of the atoms and pull the toxins out of the body.

You simply put your feet into warm water and sit there for 30 minutes. Afterward, your feet feel refreshed, just as if you had walked on a warm beach.

Your feet feel good, but what are the other benefits? You start out with clear, clean water and you end up with very ugly water. These are toxins, eliminated through your feet! Your feet are the ideal body part to release toxins -- they contain over 250,000 sweat glands and each can excrete toxins.

The color of the water can tell you the source of the toxins:

Yellow/green - urinary tract
Brown - liver and cellular debris
Dark green – gallbladder
White foam - lymphatic system
Red flecks - blood clot particles

Orange - joints
Black - liver
Cheese like particles - yeast
Black flecks - heavy metals

Parasites can also be found in the water.

The foot de-tox works on the principle of reflexology. The machine produces energy ions, positive and negative. As these ions are released, they penetrate the feet and travel through the body, bonding with the toxins and pulling them out of the body and into the water.

My machine has dual polarity to produce the negative and positive ions. During your 30-minute treatment, it switches between modes, and can even sense which ions you may need more of. For example, today you may need more positive ions to de-tox, but tomorrow you may need more negative ions.

My treatments include the foot cleanse and the infrared charcoal belt. This belt promotes better blood circulation and aids the de-tox. It also produces heat, and is comforting and relaxing.

Before your treatment, you may need to drink something like Gatorade. This type of drink contains electrolytes, and can prevent a feeling of dizziness or weakness.

The health benefits are many -- I can't list them all here, but people who suffer from *candida*, irritable bowel syndrome, trouble with memory, migraines, allergies, acne and arthritis pain may benefit most.

IRIDOLOGY

Iridology is the study of the eye or, more particularly, the iris of the eye. Iridology is a safe, non-invasive, diagnostic technique - no needles or drugs.

We look for patterns, colors, and other characteristics within the eye to determine information about a person's health. The iris is divided into zones, which correspond to certain parts of the body. Everything that is going on within your body is recorded in the eye. Even some events in the past that you may have "recovered from" are there. For instance, a surgery will be noted in the eye, no matter when you had it.

Iridology seems new to us, but has actually been around for a long time, dating back as far as 1665. It became known as *eye diagnosis* in the 19th century. Ignaz von Peczely, a Hungarian physician, accidentally broke an owl's leg as a boy, and noticed that a spot appeared in its eye at the time of the break. He nursed the owl back to health, and watched as the spot disappeared. Later, when he became a physician, he started watching the eyes of his patients. Here, again, he noticed the marks in the eye, and began making notes. Thus modern iridology was born.

In the 1950's, Bernard Jensen, an American Chiropractor, brought iridology to light in the United States. He has written many books on the subject, and is known as the Father of Iridology. He has passed his legacy on to Ellen Tart Jensen, who now carries on his work and teaches many classes on the subject.

Some iridologists use a magnifying glass and flashlight or a camera. I have a camera that takes a picture that I can run through the computer, to analyze it. I generally prefer the camera, because some people are sensitive to a light in their eyes.

But, although the camera is great, sometimes you just have to use the magnifying glass and flashlight. Your eye has layers and when looking for problems in the body, you need to know which layer of the eye it has progressed to. The layers are different colors, showing how long you have had the problem and how severe it has become. This is where the flashlight comes in handy.

You can try this yourself - take a flashlight and shine it in your eye at the side and you will see the different layers in your eye.

The eye is directly connected to the brain by the optic nerve, in direct correspondence with the brain at all times. If you look at the optic nerve, it's a mass of nerves all leading directly to the brain.

Through the brain, all of these nerve endings are linked to the various organs of the body. This is what makes the eyes the "window to the soul."

The iris can reveal many things, such as your constitution, inherent weaknesses, how you treat your body and your level of health.

The constitution is revealed in the fibers of the eye. Looking into the eye, you'll see that there are thousands of fibers present in any eye, and they have different characteristics. For instance, if the fibers are close-knit and numerous, generally you have a strong constitution, but if the fibers have space between them, it may be weaker.

With the use of Iridology you can sometimes see changes within the iris before physical symptoms develop. Then preventive action may be taken and disease avoided. The iris will reflect the condition of the tissues within the body and will show inflammation, congested lymph, acidity, hardened arteries, etc.

When looking into an iris we are not concerned with specific diseases but the conditions that set you up for disease.

For instance, cancer will not show up in the iris, but the toxicity, congestion and the level of functioning of an organ will, indicating that you have the potential for cancer. Pregnancy is something that will not show up in the eye, as it is a natural state.

To sum it up, iridology is a wonderful tool for looking at the body and determining the various states of health. Whether you use a camera or a flashlight, it can reveal valuable information about the inner workings of your body.

EAR CANDLING

This is an old practice that has been around for many years. I'm sure you have all heard of "blowing smoke in a baby's ear" as treatment for ear infections. Basically, this will do the same thing. The ear candles are strips of muslin dipped in beeswax and rolled into cones. The candle is placed in the ear and its outer edge lit; as it burns it creates a vacuum which draws out the wax buildup and toxins out of the ear. It will pull toxins out of the sinuses and Eustachian tubes. The heat will penetrate your head and is *very* relaxing.

Of course, modern medicine is really against this procedure. They throw up all kinds of cautions and dangers. Personally, I have had this done many, many times and have suffered no ill effects from it. As a matter of fact, it cleared my Eustachian tubes and stopped the infection when nothing else worked.

Several of my clients have had such good results from it, they have learned how to do it themselves and always keep candles on hand.

PARAFFIN ARTHRITIS TREATMENT

Paraffin wax treatments have been used for decades. Paraffin has been used as preservative for foods, and as a beauty treatment, but it is also very effective in treating arthritis pain. You can take these treatments daily if you need to.

I like to use the scented wax, because you'll also have aromatherapy benefits. If you use essential oils, you can gain benefits from their use as well.

The wax is heated to approximately 125°. You can mix-in a little mineral oil to keep the wax from sticking to your hands. I provide a glove, but if you are to gain benefit from essential oil, you shouldn't use it.

You submerge your hand/hands (or feet) in the warm paraffin bath, and let the wax form a layer of coating over the skin. Once the skin is coated, the paraffin will begin to dry, producing a cooling effect. Dip again after the wax dries, to form a double coat. Next, wrap the hands in a towel to contain the heat, and relax for about 20 minutes. Then just peel off the wax and you are finished.

This treatment really helps with the stiffness and pain associated with arthritis or fibromyalgia.

Paraffin treatments will increase the blood circulation, which will give the skin a healthy, glowing look.

WELLNESS/LIFE COACH

A wellness/life coach is a consultant who can provide information for living a prevention-oriented, healthy lifestyle through targeted motivational sessions. It's kind of like having a partner, by your side, to help you achieve your goals... Those goals may be better general health, stopping smoking, losing weight, etc., or they may be spiritual, emotional, or job-related.

Together, we develop a plan and have regular sessions to help you stay on track. It is similar to a basketball team hiring a coach to help them improve their game. A wellness/life coach helps you improve the game of Life -- sometimes a teacher, sometimes an encourager. We don't tell you what to do – we show you how to incorporate healthy habits into your life.

Through encouragement and empowerment, you discover the choices that are most appropriate for you and your situation. Clients are helped to identify goals, plan strategies and create structures, as well as explore underlying beliefs that may be getting in the way of their health goals.   Each case is very individual and no matter what the issue we can develop a plan to get you on track.

ZYTO BALANCE

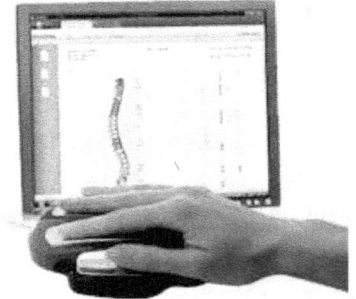

Talk about simple. It doesn't come any easier than this.

The balance is a hand-cradle, similar to a mouse for a computer. You simply rest your hand on the cradle and relax. After about 5 minutes you have a printout of your body's responses. It uses technology similar to a lie-detector test to read your responses. The cradle emits small electrical pulses through your hand and your body answers back.

From your body's answers to these pulses, we can learn a lot. It measures the functions or energy available in each organ. By tapping into your energy system, the computer and hand-cradle perform what is called a bio-survey. This consists of a sequence of computer-generated signals that are communicated to your body. To each signal, you respond, and the hand-cradle reads that response. Basically, it asks your body a question and the body answers.

At the end of the bio-survey, you can see what supplements or nutriceuticals your body responded most favorably to. This procedure actually takes the guesswork out of which supplements to choose for a healthier you. If you know what your body prefers, you can make smarter decisions about your investment in supplements. You'll save money because you'll be taking only what your body needs. And you'll improve your chances of *not getting sick in the first place*, and/or cutting down the time it takes to get better.

This Zyto technology is the most recent development by Vaughn R. Cook, OMD, who has specialized in energy medicine for the last two-and-a-half decades. It may sound like new technology, but it has a long and successful history. The Zyto Balance has been vouched-for by hundreds of thousands of patients over the past five years.

It can help you to quit shooting in the dark, and hit the bull's eye.

REIKI

Reiki is defined as a treatment in which healing energy is channeled from the practitioner to the client. This enhances patient energy and reduces pain, fatigue and stress.

Reiki was developed in 1922 by Japanese Buddhist Mikao Usui and is classified as Oriental medicine. There are two main branches of Reiki - Traditional Japanese Reiki and Western Reiki. Each form of Reiki has three degrees - First, Second and Master/Teacher degree.

Reiki is something very new to my practice and I am still learning about this very effective form of energy healing.

PULLING IT ALL TOGETHER

Your body knows instinctively what to do to make itself well. We all need to learn to listen to our bodies.

Our bodies need many things to survive in this unhealthy world. We are faced with having to take supplements instead of being able to rely on food to furnish us with what we need for optimal health. Luckily, there are good-quality supplements out there -- we may just have to look a little closer. Learn how to read labels, don't blindly trust that a supplement is high quality, and check for yourself.

A hair analysis is a very good resource for testing your mineral levels and also your toxic elements, and other natural-health techniques can help you on your way.

The plants and herbs have a signature. I believe that, if you study the shape and texture of a plant, it may give you a clue about which part of the body it will benefit. In the Appendix that comes next are more thoughts about this.

Take some responsibility for your health – you'll be glad you did. No one knows you better than you do!

Stay Strong and Healthy!

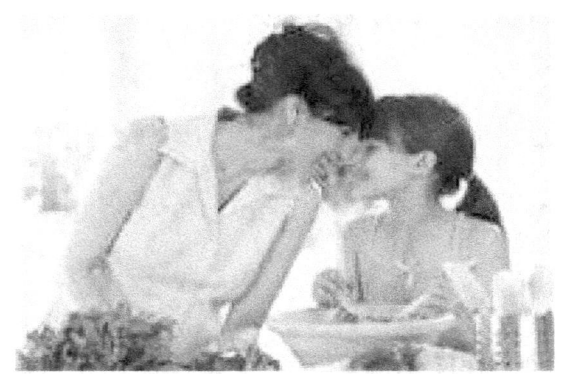

APPENDIX

An Unknown Email

This is an email I received, and it is so true that I wanted to include it in this book. I don't know who wrote it or where it came from, but it is very good. The writer clearly believes in the "Doctrine of Signatures," an ancient teaching that has survived in many parts of the globe. Today, modern science rejects it, but I think there is value in it.

"Plants, along with herbs have a signature. If we study the plant, or herb, we can tell by looking, what part of the body it will help. God left us great clues as to what foods help what part of our body! "

"A sliced Carrot looks like the human eye. The pupil, iris and radiating lines look just like the human eye... And YES, science now shows carrots greatly enhance blood flow to and function of the eyes.

"A Tomato has four chambers and is red. The heart has four chambers and is red. All of the research shows tomatoes are loaded with lycopine and are indeed pure heart and blood food.

"Grapes hang in a cluster that has the shape of the heart. Each grape looks like a blood cell and all of the research today shows grapes are also profound heart and blood vitalizing food.

"A Walnut looks like a little brain, a left and right hemisphere, upper cerebrums and lower cerebellums. Even the wrinkles or folds on the nut are just like the neo-cortex. We now know walnuts help develop more than three (3) dozen neuron-transmitters for brain function.

"Kidney Beans actually heal and help maintain kidney function and yes, they look exactly like the human kidneys.

"Celery, Bok Choy, Rhubarb and many more look just like bones. These foods specifically target bone strength. Bones are 23% sodium and these foods are 23% sodium. If you don't have enough sodium in your diet, the body pulls it from the bones, thus making them weak. These foods replenish the skeletal needs of the body.

"Avocadoes, Eggplant and Pears target the health and function of the womb and cervix of the female - they look just like these organs. Today's research shows that when a woman eats one avocado a week, it balances hormones, sheds unwanted birth weight, and prevents cervical cancers.

"Sweet Potatoes look like the pancreas and actually balance the glycemic index of diabetics.

"Figs are full of seeds and hang in twos when they grow. Figs increase the mobility of male sperm and increase the numbers of Sperm as well to overcome male sterility.

"Olives assist the health and function of the ovaries.

"Oranges, Grapefruits, and other Citrus fruits look just like the mammary glands of the female and actually assist the health of the breasts and the movement of lymph in and out of the breasts.

"Onions look like the body's cells. Today's research shows onions help clear waste materials from all of the body cells. They even produce tears which wash the epithelial layers of the eyes. A working companion, Garlic, also helps eliminate waste materials and dangerous free radicals from the body."

"And how profound is this? It takes exactly nine (9) months to grow an avocado from blossom to ripened fruit. There are over 14,000 photolytic chemical constituents of nutrition in each one of these foods (modern science has only studied and named about 141 of them)."

§

Well, that was my email. I don't know who wrote it or how long it has been circulating the internet, but it contains valuable information. Make sure you incorporate some of these foods into you next meal. You will feel much better for it!

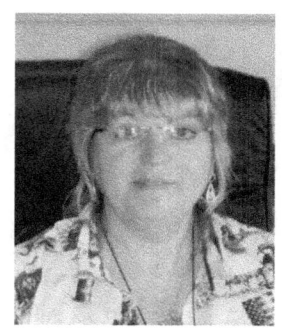

ABOUT THE AUTHOR

Dr. Sheila Miles is a native of South Central Kentucky, and grew up with a deep understanding of culture, tradition, and the many intangibles that make us who we are. She also saw close-to-hand a wide spectrum of health problems, and the ways country people had learned to deal with them, sometimes because a doctor was not available, and sometimes because the natural ways were better than the doctors'.

While coping with normal health issues involved in raising her own family, Sheila realized that she could help them better, and help her community as well, by learning more about natural medicine.

She went back to school, and in 2000 was Board Certified as a Naturopathic Physician by the National Board of Examiners in Integrated/Alternative Medicine and Natural Health Science. In addition, she earned a Doctorate in Natural Health Science.

Dr. Miles is certified in Iridology, Manipulation, Hydrotherapy, Acupressure Massage, Nutrition, Homeopathy, and Herbal Preparations, and as a Life Coach and a NLP practitioner.

She feels a strong mission to help wherever possible, using the natural medical practices that work in harmony with our own systems to bring about natural health.